HOW TO TALK TO KIDS ABOUT NUTRITION

Practical Parenting Tips to Tackle Picky Eaters, Minimise Processed Foods, and Boost Their Immune Systems while Making it Fun

CLEMMIE PELLEW-HARVEY, dipNT mBANT

Pownall
Publishing

Photography: Emma Webb Photography

First edition

For Pia,

My sweet girl, my greatest achievement. Thank you for making me a mother and for inspiring me to step out of my comfort zone to write this book. This journey wouldn't have been possible without you.

Love

Mummy x

FREE
Bonus Pack

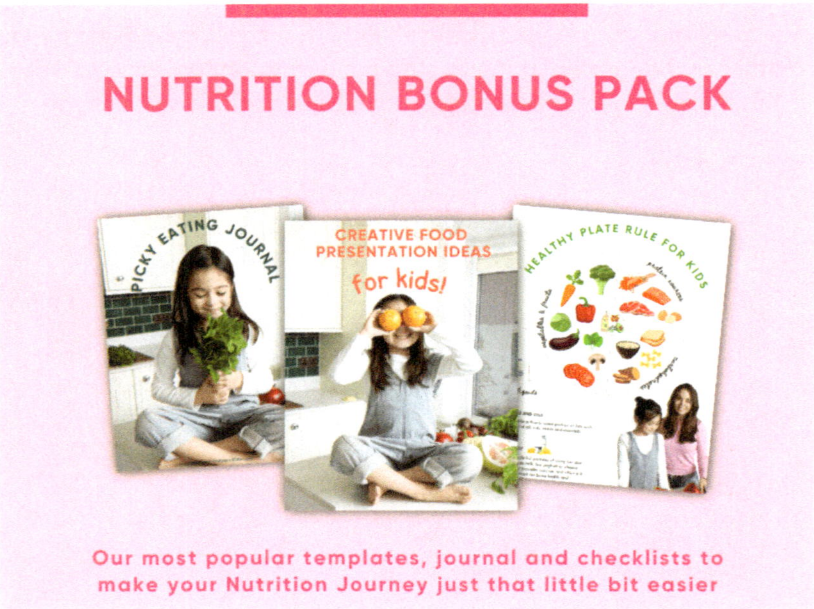

Join our VIP Review Panel and get this detailed Nutrition Tools Bundle for FREE.

To download it:

- If you are on Kindle then click click the image above
- Otherwise simply use your phone to scan the QR code

SCAN ME!

Contents

Introduction

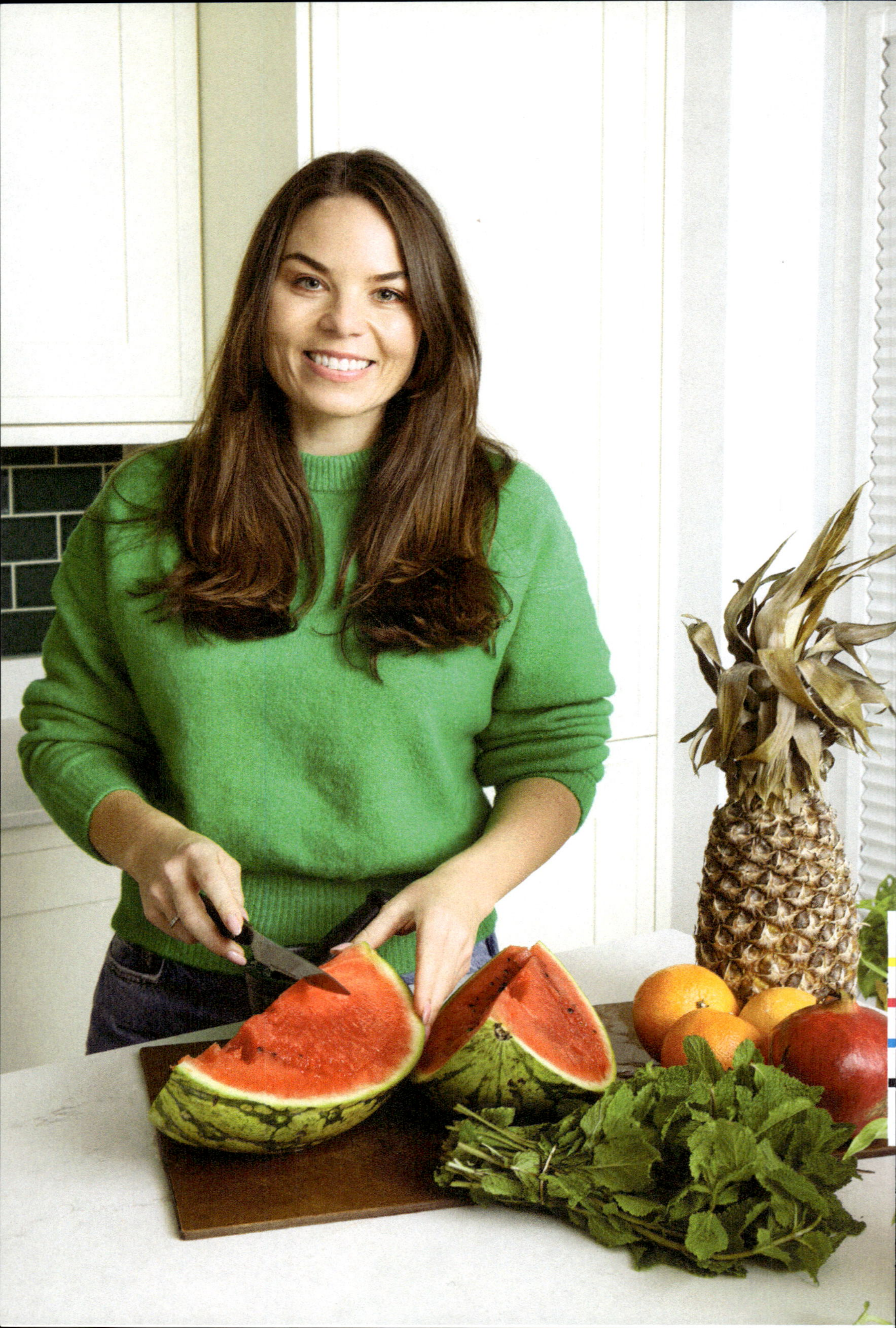

Introduction

I'm in the kitchen, trying to prevent my daughter from grabbing yet another snack. Dinner isn't going according to plan, and she's adamant about having cheesy pasta again. Meanwhile, I can't shake off the thought of all the snacks she's already had since school pick-up. Time is running out, and I'm trying to figure out how to put something healthy on the table while also ensuring she eats something. Does this sound familiar to you?

Many mothers face the same challenges when it comes to feeding their kids. Picky eaters are a common hurdle. It's hard not to rely on quick and convenient processed foods. Yet, deep down, we all want our kids to eat well and stay healthy. Studies show that nearly 50% of parents say their child is a picky eater. Many also worry about their child's immune health and the long-term effects of their diet.

There's a lot at stake here, and it goes far beyond just food. It's about nurturing a healthy relationship with what we eat. The link between a lack of nutrition education and the growing number of eating disorders is undeniable. The statistics are staggering—around 30 million people in the U.S. will face an eating disorder at some point in their lives. As parents, it's our responsibility to help our children develop a positive mindset around food and body image. It starts with us, and it's crucial that we lead by example, showing them a balanced, healthy approach to eating.

That's where I come in. I'm Clementine Pellew-Harvey, but you can call me Clemmie. As a Nutritional Therapist and a mum, I understand these struggles firsthand. I trained at the College of Naturopathic Medicine and have worked with a wide range of people, from high-profile clients to families like yours. I also collaborate with The Kyros Project at Google DeepMind, helping people gain insights into their health through advanced biomedical testing. It's a bit ironic that, despite my background, I have a picky eater at home. However, this experience has reinforced the importance of making nutrition fun and accessible, ultimately inspiring me to write this book!

During a recent visit with my daughter Pia's godmother, I asked Pia what she'd like to eat, and her response was classic: "Cheesy pasta, pizza, chips, ketchup, and chicken nuggets." A nutritionist's dream, right? Her family chuckled and mentioned how comforting it was to hear that Pia still enjoys these kinds of foods. And that's exactly the essence of this book – it's not about transforming your child into the "perfect" eater (because there's no such thing). Yes, I'm a nutritionist, but I'm also a mum, and beige food still finds its way onto Pia's plate.

This book is designed to equip kids with the knowledge they'll need as they grow, empowering them to make balanced, healthy choices for themselves in the long run. It's not about perfection; it's about progress. My vision is straightforward: to provide you with the tools and understanding to make healthy eating a reality for your family. We'll explore nutrition from two angles: first, understanding what healthy eating truly means, and second, making it enjoyable for your kids. Together, we'll create a balanced approach to food that your children can carry with them for life.

You, the busy mum in your late 20s to early 40s, are exactly who I'm talking to! I know you're on the hunt for practical solutions to elevate your child's diet without adding to your stress levels. You want simple tips that fit seamlessly into your chaotic life because, let's face it, who has time for elaborate meal prep when you're juggling work deadlines, school pick-ups, homework and a toddler insisting on being your little shadow?

Here's what you can expect from this book: we're diving straight into the picky eating battleground with tried-and-true strategies that have worked wonders for me and many others. We'll explore fun ways to get your kids involved in the kitchen as well as tackling dietary restrictions, helping you navigate them like a pro. And yes, we'll discuss when supplementation might be useful—because sometimes even the best intentions need a bit of extra support!

What makes this book truly special? It's packed with personal stories and tips that have been tested in real family kitchens, mine included! You'll find interactive elements to keep you and your little ones engaged, along with a variety of recipes and cultural insights that cater to diverse tastes and backgrounds.

I'd like to set some clear expectations. This book offers actionable advice and realistic goals. It's all about creating a healthier eating environment at home but remember: change doesn't happen overnight. It's like trying to teach your kids to share their toys- small, consistent steps can lead to significant improvements in your family's health.

CLEMMIE'S Tip

You can see some of my thinking about my approach in this short video on my YouTube channel or scan the QR code

I'd love for you to join me on this journey toward better nutrition and a happier relationship with food. And if you ever feel like you need some one-on-one advice or support, don't hesitate to reach out. I'm here for you! Plus, if you have any helpful tips of your own, I'm all ears!

CLEMMIE'S Tip

I've set up a dedicated Private Facebook Group for readers of this book, "How To Talk To Kids About Nutrition Group", where parents can share tips, ideas, stories, and ask whatever is on their mind. We share advice, new recipes, supplier discounts and much more. Come and check us out and join in the conversation!

Join the dedicated Facebook group or scan the QR code.

Here's to making a real difference in your family's well-being, one meal at a time, with a side of fun!

Chapter One

Understanding the Basics of Child Nutrition

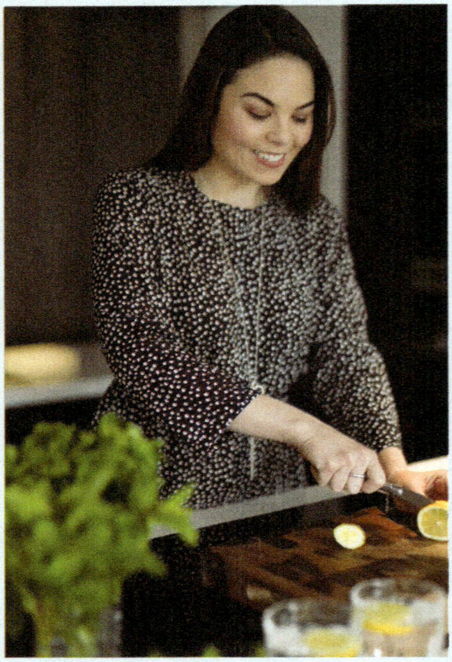
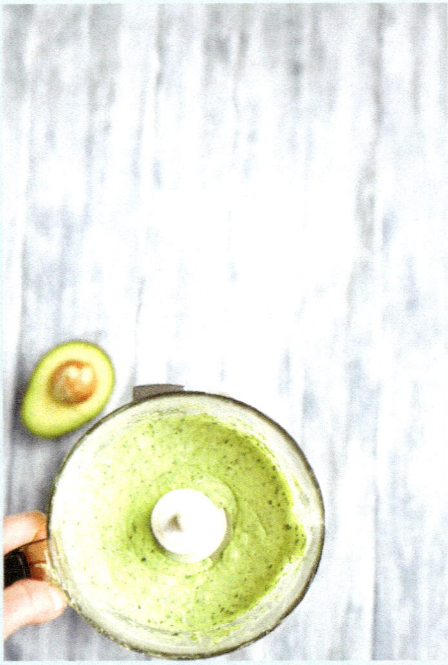
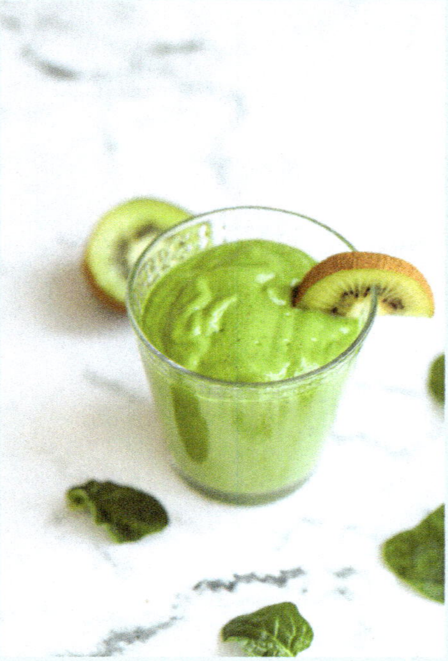
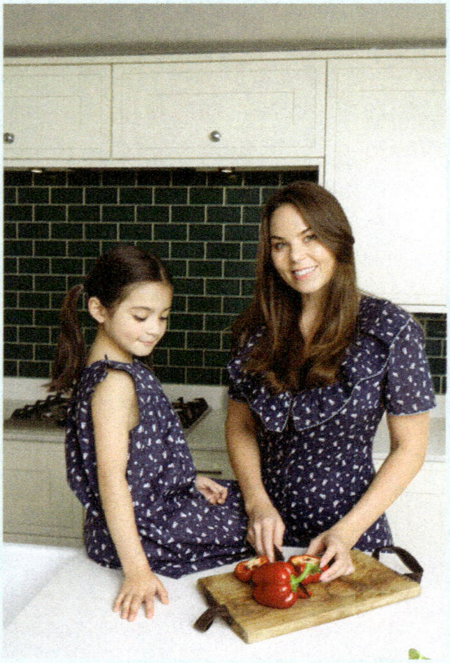

Understanding the Basics of Child Nutrition

Have you ever watched your little one pick through their plate, happily munching on pasta while the broccoli sits untouched? I know that scene all too well with Pia - she's still not a massive fan unless I sneak it in somehow, though she'll eat the stalks, which I'll gladly take!

As mums, we all want our kids to eat what's good for them, but it can feel like an uphill battle. You might wonder if they're getting enough nutrients to grow up strong and healthy. It's a worry many of us share, especially when life gets busy and convenience takes over. But knowing exactly what nutrients they need can ease those worries and help you feel confident in the meals you're putting on the table. Let's dive into the essentials together.

Nutrients Kids Need: A Breakdown

Children thrive on a diet rich in essential nutrients, each critical to their growth and development. Protein is the fundamental building block vital for muscle growth and repair. Think of it as the scaffolding that helps your child build strong muscles and a robust immune system. Lean meats, beans, and legumes are excellent sources of protein. These foods pack a punch without the added fats, making them ideal for little bodies that are growing rapidly and need all the support they can get.

Calcium and Vitamin D are partners in crime when it comes to bone health. They're the dynamic duo that ensures your child develops strong bones and teeth. Dairy products like milk and yoghurt are classic sources, but don't overlook fortified plant milks. These are fantastic alternatives, especially if your household leans towards a plant-based diet. They ensure your child gets the necessary nutrients without compromising their dietary preferences or needs.

Iron is another powerhouse nutrient, crucial for healthy blood cells and energy levels. It's what keeps your child lively and enthusiastic, ready to take on the world or at least the playground. Red meat, spinach, and lentils are iron-rich options. Remember, pairing iron-rich foods with a source of vitamin C, such as oranges or strawberries, can enhance absorption.

Then there's omega-3 fatty acids, often hailed as brain food. These nutrients support cognitive development and mental health, fueling your child's growing brain. Fish such as salmon, walnuts, and flaxseeds are packed with these beneficial fats. Including them in your child's diet can aid in everything from concentration to overall mood, helping them excel both in school and social settings.

Flaxseed and walnut energy ball recipe (see opposite)

CLEMMIE'S Tip

Quick and easy walnut flax energy bites. These little walnut bites are a good source of plant-based omega-3 and fiber. Keep them in the freezer for a quick nutritious snack!

Check our recipes on our YouTube channel or scan the QR code

While these nutrients are crucial, it's essential to recognise the foods that offer the most nutritional bang for your buck. Dark leafy greens like kale and Swiss chard are nutrient-dense champions. They're low in calories but high in vitamins, minerals, and fibre. Whole grains such as quinoa and brown rice are also excellent choices, providing sustained energy and supporting digestive health. Don't forget about berries, such as blueberries and strawberries, which are brimming with antioxidants that protect your child's body from environmental stressors.

Despite our best efforts, some deficiencies are still common in children. Vitamin D deficiency, for instance, often rears its head during the winter months when sunlight is scarce. Iron deficiency can be a concern, particularly in vegetarian diets. Fortified foods can help bridge these gaps. By choosing products fortified with these nutrients, you can help ensure your child gets what they need to thrive.

Understanding these basics helps you make informed choices. You can create meals that are not only nutritious but also enjoyable for your child. Whether it's sneaking spinach into a stew or offering a variety of colourful fruits, every small

FLAXSEED AND WALNUT ENERGY BALLS

Prep: 15 Mins Chill: 15 mins

Makes 20 Balls

- 1 cup rolled oats
- 1/2 cup ground flaxseed
- 1/2 cup walnuts, finely chopped (or any nut of your choice)
- 1/3 cup honey or maple syrup
- 1/2 cup nut butter (peanut, almond, or sunflower seed butter)
- 1/4 cup mini chocolate chips or dried fruit (optional)
- 1 teaspoon vanilla extract
- Pinch of salt (optional)

Quick and easy walnut flax energy bites. These little walnut bites are a good source of plant-based omega-3 and fiber. Keep them in the freezer for a quick nutritious snack! a nutritious snack that kids will love, packed with healthy fats, fibre, and a touch of sweetness!

Instructions

In a large mixing bowl, combine the rolled oats, ground flaxseed, chopped walnuts, and a pinch of salt if using.

In a separate bowl, mix together the honey (or maple syrup), nut butter, and vanilla extract until smooth.

Pour the wet mixture into the dry ingredients and stir until everything is well combined. If using chocolate chips or dried fruit, fold them in at this stage.

Using your hands, scoop out small amounts of the mixture and roll them into balls about 1 inch in diameter.

Place the energy balls on a baking sheet or plate and refrigerate for at least 30 minutes to firm up.

CLEMMIE'S Tip

Keep the energy balls in an airtight container in the refrigerator for up to a week. They also freeze well, so you can make a batch ahead of time!

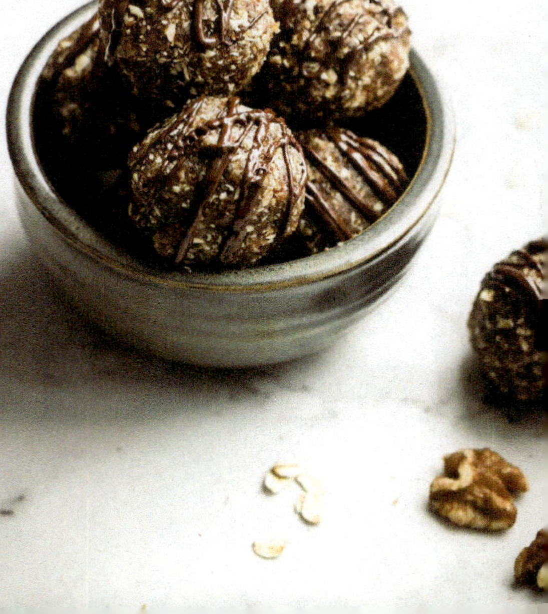

step counts in building a foundation for lifelong health.

Building Balanced Meals: The Plate Method

Imagine a plate made just for picky eaters, where half is filled with foods they already love and are familiar with, such as carrots and peas, a quarter with a protein they enjoy or will at least have some of, and the last bit with a familiar starch or grain. It keeps things simple and helps create balanced meals without all the second-guessing. In our house, for example, I might put together some cut-up chicken with a small serving of pasta, plus a few carrot sticks or cucumber slices (Pia loves those!). Or, I'll try sneaking in some veggies by making a pasta dish loaded with my go-to 'Hulk' sauce (recipe below) and a generous sprinkle of cheese.

If I've made rice, I'll pair it with some homemade fish goujons (recipe below) and let her choose a mild vegetable she's comfortable with. The goal is to offer a good mix of nutrients without overwhelming them. And let me tell you, cheese has always been a saviour in our house; I'm definitely not above using it as a bribe to introduce new foods!

Home-made Fish Goujon Recipe

CLEMMIE'S Tip

Quick and easy homemade fish fingers that are always popular and bursting with nutrients! These are so much better than shop bought fish-fingers and so much healthier.

Check our recipes on our YouTube channel or scan the QR code

Hulk Sauce Recipe

CLEMMIE'S Tip

This vibrant green Hulk sauce is not only delicious but also packed with nutrients, making it a perfect accompaniment for pasta or with any meat!

Check our recipes on our YouTube channel or scan the QR code

It's important to remember that what works for one age group might not suit another. For toddlers, small portions with more frequent meals tend to work better. Their tiny tummies can only handle so much at once, so spreading out their meals

HOMEMADE FISH GOUJONS

Prep: 15 Mins Cook: 20 mins

Serves 2

2 fillets of white fish (like cod, haddock, or pollock)

1 cup whole wheat breadcrumbs (or panko for extra crunch)

1/2 cup plain flour

1 large egg

1 teaspoon garlic powder

1 teaspoon paprika

Salt and pepper to taste

1 tablespoon olive oil (for baking)

Quick and easy homemade fish fingers that are always popular and bursting with nutrients!

Instructions

Preheat your oven to 200°C (400°F) and line a baking sheet with parchment paper.

Set up three bowls: one with flour (seasoned with salt and pepper), one with beaten egg, and one with breadcrumbs mixed with garlic powder and paprika.

Cut the fish fillets into strips (about 1 inch wide).

Dip each fish strip first into the flour, shaking off excess.

Next, dip into the beaten egg, letting any excess drip off.

Finally, coat in the breadcrumb mixture, pressing lightly to adhere.

Place the coated fish strips on the prepared baking sheet and drizzle with olive oil.

Bake in the preheated oven for about 15-20 minutes, or until golden brown and cooked through

CLEMMIE'S Tip

Serve with the Homemade Hulk sauce. Delicious!

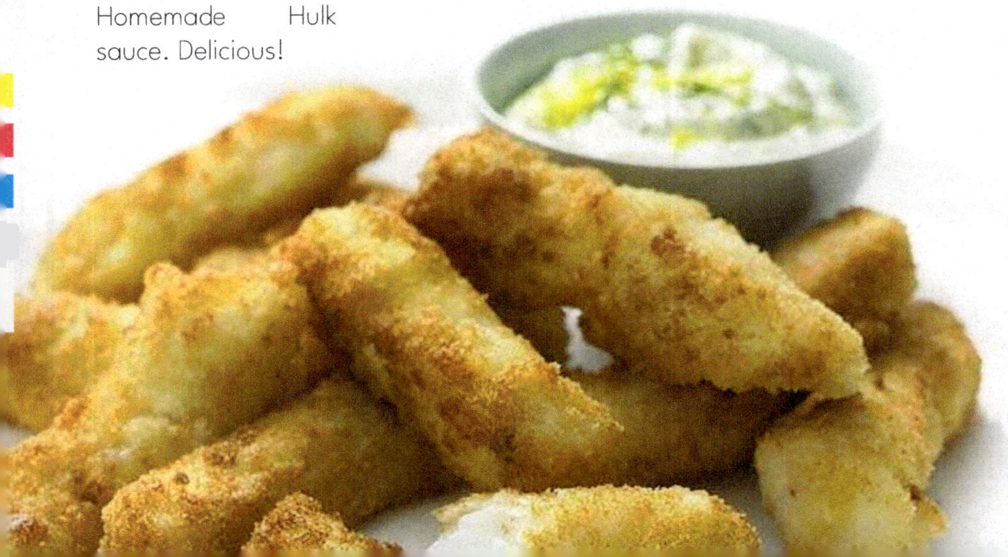

HULK SAUCE

Prep: 15 Mins

Serve 6

1 ripe avocado

1 cup fresh spinach leaves

1/4 cup fresh herbs (like parsley, coriander, or basil)

1/4 cup grated cheese (such as cheddar or feta)

1 tablespoon lemon juice

Salt and pepper to taste

This vibrant green Hulk sauce is not only delicious but also packed with nutrients, making it a perfect accompaniment for pasta or with any meat!

Instructions

Blend Ingredients: In a blender or food processor, combine the avocado, spinach, fresh herbs, grated cheese, and lemon juice.

Season: Add salt and pepper to taste, then blend until smooth and creamy.

Serve: Transfer the Hulk sauce to a fun dipping bowl and enjoy it with the homemade fish goujons!

This vibrant green Hulk sauce is not only delicious but also packed with nutrients, making it a perfect accompaniment for pasta or with any meat

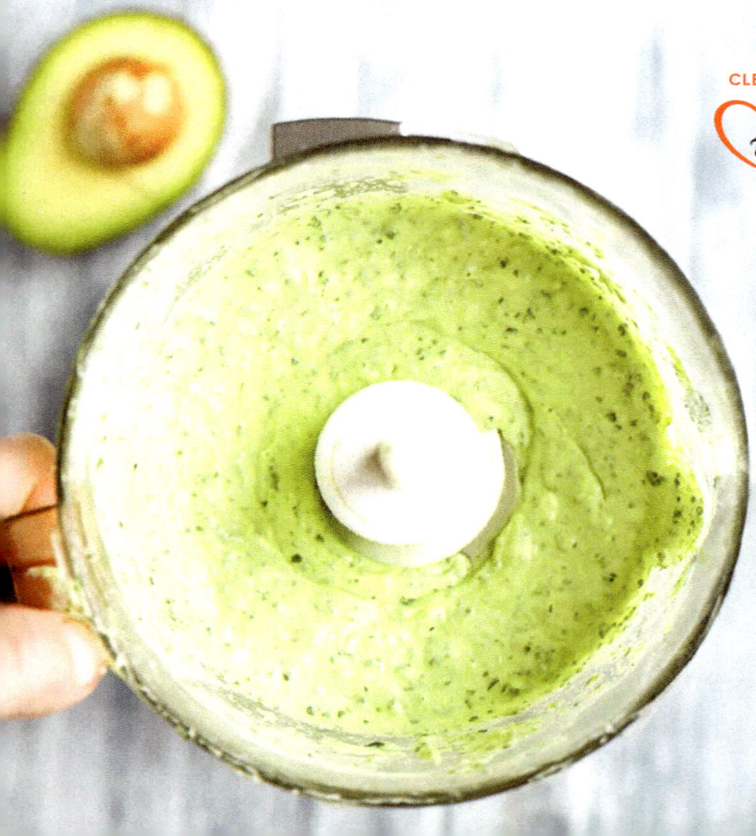

CLEMMIE'S Tip

Great with Fish Goujons or even just as a dip on ts own,

helps keep energy levels steady. In contrast, active school-aged kids might need more protein and complex carbohydrates to fuel their busy days. Think of how different a toddler's plate looks compared to a teenager's, and adjust accordingly. The same method applies, just with tweaks to portion sizes and frequency.

There's also the matter of cultural and dietary preferences. The beauty of the plate method is its adaptability. For families following a vegetarian or vegan diet, lentils or beans can serve as the protein source. These can be as satisfying and nutritious as meat. Similarly, traditional grains such as millet or bulgar wheat can replace rice, adding variety and cultural richness to meals. These adjustments ensure that the plate method doesn't just cater to one type of diet. It's flexible enough to incorporate the diverse dietary practices found in households worldwide.

Visual Guide: Create Your Own Plate

Draw a circle and divide it into sections. Label one-half "vegetables and fruits," one-quarter "protein," and the remaining quarter "grains." Fill in each section with meal ideas you know your child loves. This can be a fun fridge activity to do together.

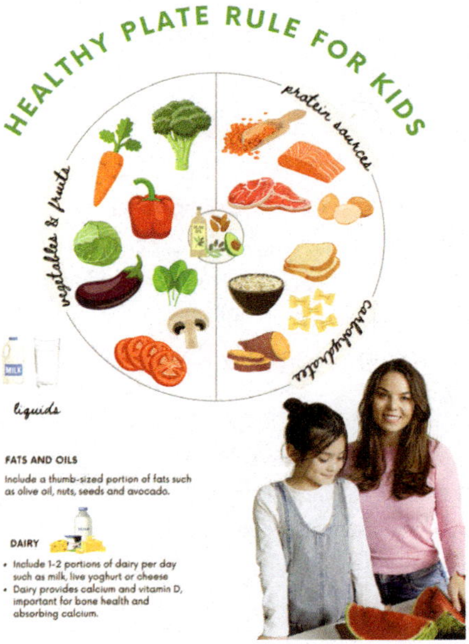

Through these small, thoughtful steps, you can build balanced meals that are both nutritious and appealing. The plate method offers a straightforward way to visualise and plan meals. It helps make healthy eating more accessible and less of a chore.

Your free copy of the Visual Plate guide is included in the bonus pack which you can download from the link and QR code at the front of the book.

Reading Food Labels: Decoding Ingredients

You've ventured out for a food shop, list in hand, trying to make the best choices for your family's health. You're surrounded by aisles packed with options, each promising something better than the last. But how do you cut through the noise? It all starts with reading food labels, a skill that's more powerful than you might think.

Nutrition Facts Valeur nutritive Per 1 cup (250 mL) / par 1 tasse (250 mL)	
Amount Teneur	**% Daily Value % valeur quotidienne**
Calories / Calories 80	
Fat / Lipides 0 g	0 %
Saturated / saturés 0 g + Trans / trans 0 g	0 %
Cholesterol / Cholestérol 0 mg	
Sodium / Sodium 115 mg	5 %
Carbohydrate / Glucides 12 g	4 %
Fibre / Fibres 0 g	0 %
Sugars / Sucres 11 g	
Protein / Protéines 9 g	
Vitamin A / Vitamine A	15 %
Vitamin C / Vitamine C	0 %
Calcium / Calcium	30 %
Iron / Fer	0 %
Vitamin D / Vitamine D	45 %

Understanding these labels can transform how you shop, giving you the confidence to choose foods that are genuinely good for your family. It begins with serving sizes. Often, what seems like a single portion is actually two or more servings. This detail affects the entire nutrition profile on that label. Knowing this can help you gauge how much you and your family are really consuming. Then, there are calories and macronutrients (proteins, carbs, and fats) that fuel our bodies. Monitor these to ensure each choice aligns with your dietary goals and needs.

The ingredient list is another critical section, especially for spotting allergens or unwanted additives. Here, manufacturers must list ingredients in descending order by weight, so the first few items are what you're primarily consuming. Be wary of long lists with unrecognisable names. These often indicate a heavily processed product. Allergen information is usually highlighted, but it's worth double-checking, especially if your child has specific dietary needs.

Spotting hidden sugars and additives can feel like detective work. Sugar hides under many aliases like high fructose corn syrup, sucrose, and glucose. Recognising these can be a game-changer, especially when managing your child's sugar intake. For additives, look out for names like aspartame or sodium benzoate. These preservatives might extend a product's shelf life, but often at the expense of your family's health.

Choosing healthier options becomes easier once you know what to look for. When comparing cereals, for example, check the fibre content. Higher fibre not only aids digestion but also keeps kids feeling fuller longer. For canned goods, opt for low-sodium versions to manage salt intake without sacrificing convenience.

When I started focusing on nutrient density, it really changed how I thought about food. Instead of just looking at calories, I began paying attention to the quality of those calories. For example, fresh fruits, veggies, or whole grains pack more nutrients into every bite than processed foods. This simple shift means I'm giving Pia (and the rest of us!) the best fuel for our bodies. One trick I've found helpful is checking the daily value percentages on labels. It's an easy way to see at a glance how a food fits into a balanced diet, so you can make more intelligent choices without feeling like you need to be a nutrition expert.

At first, decoding food labels felt a bit overwhelming for me, too, but it's honestly a skill that's been so worth developing. Once I got the hang of it, I realised how much power it gave me to choose foods that genuinely support my family's health. I now take a moment to check the labels, and it's incredible what you can learn with just a quick glance. It's become second nature to me, and I feel so much more confident knowing I'm making choices that align with what we need to thrive.

Portion Sizes for Growing Bodies

Portion sizes can be so tricky, especially with labels like "small," "regular," or "large" thrown around without much thought. I've noticed how these words can really shape how we think about food, often more than we realise. When I hear "regular," I might picture a modest serving, but it could mean a much heartier plate for someone else. This difference can really affect how we feed our children and how they develop their own eating habits.

With Pia, I've learned that smaller portions are key. At 7, she's active but still benefits from meals that suit her needs without overwhelming her. As kids grow, their portion needs to change, too. School-aged children thrive on balanced meals that match their energy levels and activity. It's all about finding what works best and adjusting as they grow!

Cultural influences play a significant role in how we view portion sizes. What one family sees as a "generous helping," another might call a normal portion. You might have grown up hearing things like, "Finish everything on your plate," or even find yourself saying to your own kids, "No dessert unless you eat all your dinner." Many of us were raised with this mindset, and breaking out of it is tough.

But did you know that children are naturally quite good at knowing when they're full? Within reason, it's important to respect their hunger cues, even when it feels tricky not to push them to eat more. In many cultures, serving large portions is a way to show love and hospitality, but it can sometimes encourage overeating if we're not careful.

There are simple ways to manage portions without it feeling like a big deal. For instance, using smaller plates and bowls can help control portion sizes naturally. Teaching mindful eating habits such as pausing during meals to ask, "Am I still hungry?" can encourage kids to listen to their bodies and develop a healthier relationship with food.

The language we use around food and portions influences satiety and satisfaction. Describing a meal as "just right" can promote a sense of adequacy and contentment, guiding kids towards mindful eating. In contrast, terms like "indulgent" or "huge" may inadvertently encourage overeating. This is why using precise, appropriate language is so important. It helps teach children healthy eating habits and educates everyone about balanced nutrition. Proper portion control can play a significant role in managing weight and preventing disordered eating and chronic conditions later in life.

Marketing often manipulates language to entice us into consuming more than we need. Phrases like "jumbo" or "family size" are designed to suggest value but usually lead to overconsumption. By understanding this, you can empower yourself and your family to make informed decisions. Clear language helps you accurately interpret portion sizes, leading to more responsible choices.

Visual aids can simplify this learning process. For example, you could use a deck of cards to visualise a serving of meat or a tennis ball to gauge the right amount of grains like rice or pasta. These everyday items offer relatable comparisons, making it easier to understand and teach portion sizes to your children.

Balancing portion sizes with nutritional needs is crucial. As children grow, their activity levels and developmental stages dictate their nutritional requirements. Ensuring their protein intake matches their activity level and adjusting portions as they advance through different growth phases is essential. This balance helps meet their needs without overloading them with unnecessary calories.

Ultimately, understanding and managing portion sizes is about more than just what's on the plate. It's about shaping healthy eating habits, fostering a positive relationship with food, and empowering your family to make choices that support their well-being. With the right approach, you can help your children grow up with a balanced view of food, where they feel satisfied and nourished without the need for excess. These practices will serve them so well throughout life, laying the groundwork for a healthier, more mindful approach to eating.

What To Do Next

1. Try the plate method - fill half your plate with fruits/veggies, quarter with protein, and quarter with grains. Pop the visual guide on your fridge as a quick reminder!

2. Add omega-rich foods to your weekly shopping list —think salmon, walnuts, or seeds. They're tasty, add variety and are brilliant for growing brains!

3. Make those nutrients work harder by pairing iron-rich foods (like spinach or red meat) with vitamin C foods (pop in some strawberries or orange segments).

4. Get label-savvy! Start checking ingredient lists and spotting sneaky sugars—anything ending in 'ose' is usually sugar disguised and should be avoided, if possible.

5. Use everyday objects as portion guides - a deck of cards for meat portions or a tennis ball for pasta helps keep things simple and ensures that you don't waste anything too.

6. Stock up on calcium superstars - dairy or fortified plant milks are perfect for growing bones and can be drunk on their own or used in some of our delicious recipes

7. Give the recipes a go! Grab the ingredients for the energy balls, fish goujons or the 'Hulk' sauce and get your kids to join in the cooking.

8. Trust your little one's hunger cues. Remember, they're naturally good at knowing when they're full, even if the plate isn't empty, so take their guidance!

Chapter Two

Tackling Picky Eaters

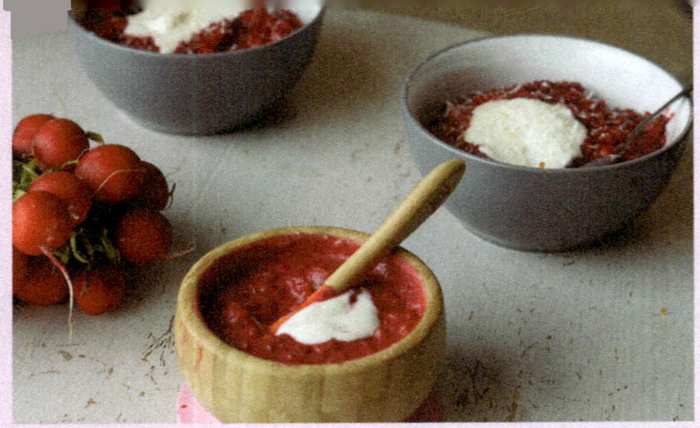

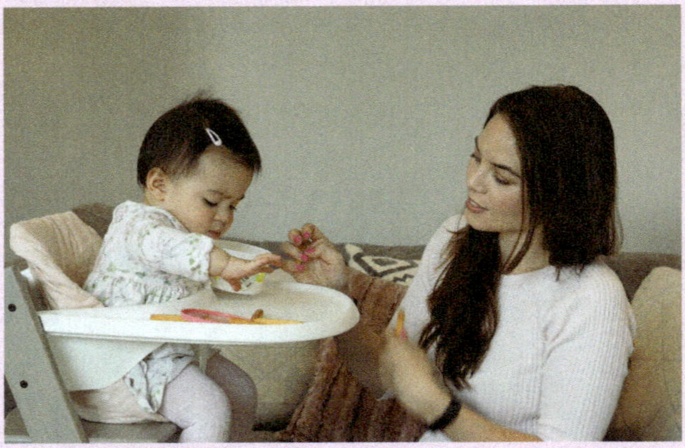

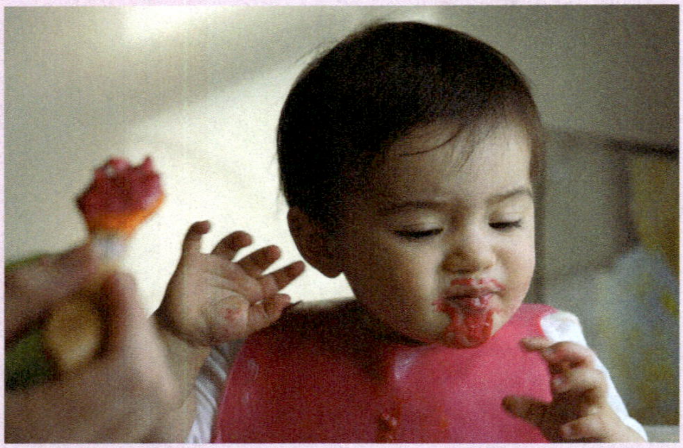

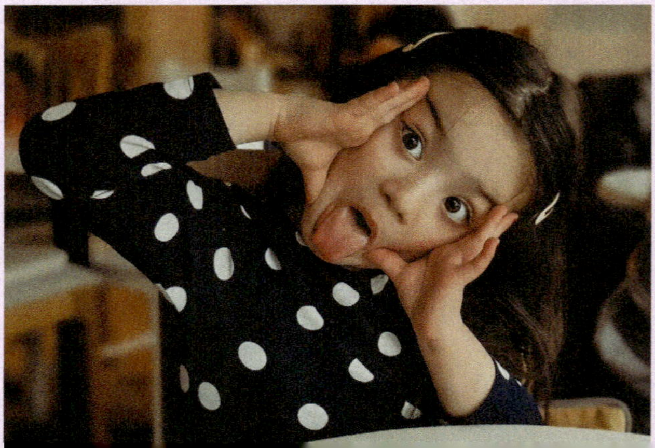

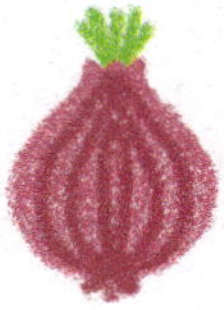

Tackling Picky Eating

It's dinnertime, and you're serving a colourful plate of sautéed vegetables and grilled chicken. Your child, however, is eyeing the plate with suspicion. They poke at the chicken as if it's a foreign object. Sound familiar?

Pia still rarely touches chicken unless it's safely hidden inside a pie or breaded. If it's just sitting there plain or, heaven forbid, is decorated with the tiniest sprinkling of herbs, game over. But hey, that doesn't stop me from trying! I'm convinced constant exposure will eventually wear her down.

Many mums have been through the picky-eating battle; it's a parenting milestone! You pour your heart into making a healthy meal, only to be met with refusal or that face from your child. It's exhausting and frustrating! But there is a silver lining: when you get a handle on the psychology behind picky eating, it can really change the game. It won't fix things instantly, but it can make mealtimes a whole lot less stressful and even a bit more fun!

At the heart of picky eating is a psychological phenomenon known as neophobia, or the fear of new foods. This is particularly common in toddlers, who are naturally cautious about unfamiliar tastes and textures. It's a developmental stage that, while challenging, is perfectly normal. Children's sensory processing plays a significant role here. Some kids are more sensitive to the textures and flavours of food, which can influence their preferences. You might notice they shy away from certain foods because they're too "mushy" or "spicy." Recognising these sensory issues is the first step in understanding your child's eating habits.

When Pia was about ten months old, I had a terrifying moment when she nearly choked on a frozen banana. It shook me so much that I only gave her blended food and pouches for months afterwards because I wanted to play it safe. I'm pretty sure that's part of why she's so sensitive to certain textures now, and I can't help but feel a little responsible for it. It's funny how those early experiences can have such a lasting impact on what our kids are picky about!

Picky eating habits can sometimes reveal deeper feelings. For instance, a child might refuse to try new foods, even when hungry, and instead reach for sweet or bland options that feel familiar and comforting. It's not just stubbornness; it's often their way of finding control or feeling secure with what they know. I can completely relate to this as an adult. Certain foods bring me immense comfort because they're connected to such fond memories. My grandma used to make the best rice pudding, and it's still my all-time favourite dessert. My mum always made us homemade weekday meals such as sausage casserole and "spag bol", and my dad's Sunday roasts were unbeatable - the common theme with all of these is that they made me feel safe and loved. Sometimes, we just need that little bit of comfort in our lives!

As parents, we have such a significant impact on how our kids approach food, even if we don't realise it. The way we act and talk about food can really shape their attitudes. When they see us enjoying different foods, it sends the message that trying new things can be fun and normal. It's tempting to use pressure or bribes to get them to eat (I'm still a little guilty of this with Pia!). But I've learned that easing up on the pressure and focusing more on praise works way better. Creating a relaxed, positive vibe around meals encourages them to explore new foods without making it a battle.

To address psychological barriers, consider strategies that gently challenge your child's reluctance. Gradual exposure techniques can be effective. Introduce new foods alongside familiar favourites, allowing your child to explore them at their own pace. Positive reinforcement works wonders, too. Praise your child for small attempts, whether they take a bite or simply touch the new food. Encouragement goes a long way in building their confidence and willingness to try.

Overcoming picky eating is not about achieving perfection. It's about creating a supportive environment where your child feels safe to explore new foods without judgment or pressure. Understanding the psychological aspects allows you to tailor your approach to meet your child's unique needs. Remember, patience and empathy are your best allies in this journey.

Gentle Introductions: New Foods, New Tastes

Introducing new foods to kids takes time and a bit of creativity. You don't need to change what's on their plate overnight completely. Instead, think of it as slowly widening their food world. Start small; if your child loves pasta, try mixing in some

Interactive Element: Picky Eating Journal

Encourage your child to keep a "Picky Eating Journal." Each week, note the foods your child has tried, how they feel about them, and what they'd like to try next. This can help track progress and make your child feel involved in their food choices.

A free PDF copy of the **Picky Eating Journal** is included in the bonus pack which you can download from the link and QR code at the front of the book.

roasted veggies or sneaking in a bit of grated carrot. The new food doesn't have to be the main focus, but with repeated exposure, they'll start to feel more comfortable with it over time. It's like making a new friend; it takes time to warm up.

One of the most delightful ways to introduce new foods is through creative presentation. Food art can transform a simple plate of veggies into a playful scene. A cucumber slice can become a smiling face, while carrot sticks might form a sun's rays. By turning mealtime into a fun activity, you can spark curiosity and engagement. Involve your child in this process, too. Let them arrange their food, creating their own edible masterpiece. This involvement not only gives them a sense of ownership but also makes them more likely to try what they've helped create.

CLEMMIE'S Tip

Your free PDF copy of the **Creative Meals Ideas** is included in the bonus pack which you can download from the link and QR code at the front of the book.

While persistence is critical, respecting your child's pace is crucial. Encouragement should be gentle, without pressure or negativity. Avoid labelling them as a "picky eater," which can reinforce unhelpful stereotypes. Instead, adopt a no-pressure tasting policy. Offer foods without demanding they eat them. A simple "Would you like to try this?" can be far more effective than a command. Such an approach fosters a more open attitude toward trying new foods, making it a choice rather than a chore. When they do take a bite, celebrate it, no matter how small. Each bite is a step forward.

One of my clients had a daughter who wanted nothing to do with anything green on her plate. I suggested they make veggies more fun, so they started serving "broccoli trees" and turned mealtime into a little adventure. What was once a food battle became something playful, and she started getting excited about her meals. Over time, she stopped avoiding the veggies and even started asking for broccoli as a snack! It just goes to show that big changes can happen with a bit of creativity and patience - even with the pickiest of eaters!

Another one of my clients had a son who was all about soft foods; anything crunchy was an absolute no-go. We took a slow and steady approach, gradually introducing different textures. They started by adding a single crunchy carrot slice alongside his favourite mashed potatoes so it didn't feel overwhelming. With a bit of patience and encouragement, he started to get more comfortable with these new textures. Eventually, his diet expanded without any drama, and crunchy foods stopped being such a big deal! It's a reminder that small, manageable changes can make a big difference over time.

These stories show how much of a difference gentle, no-pressure approaches can make with picky eaters. When you make trying new foods fun instead of stressful, it changes the whole vibe around mealtimes. It's not just about expanding your child's diet; it's about helping them build a healthy, positive relationship with food. Meals should feel like little moments of discovery and joy, where exploring new flavours becomes a regular, exciting part of their day. This approach makes it easier for everyone - kids feel less anxious, and you feel less frustrated!

Creating a Positive Mealtime Environment

For so many of us, the kitchen table is where the day's craziness starts to melt away. It's more than just a place to eat—it's where you connect with your family. This atmosphere plays a huge role in whether or not your child is open to trying new foods. Creating a routine with regular mealtimes is key because kids thrive on that predictability. Knowing that dinner is always at six, for example, gives them a sense of comfort and can ease any anxiety around food. Add to that the importance of cutting out distractions - turn off the TV, put the phones away and you've got a space where everyone is truly present. It's not just about the food; it's about sharing stories, bonding, and making mealtime something everyone looks forward to.

Family dynamics at the table are so important! Encouraging open conversations about food can help your child feel comfortable sharing what they like (or don't like) without feeling judged. It's not just about the food - it's about understanding and respecting each other's preferences. Sometimes, you'll find out that what your child dislikes isn't even about the taste but the texture! Keeping things pressure-free is key. Forget the whole "you must finish your plate" idea and instead celebrate the little wins, like trying something new. It's all about making mealtime a relaxed, enjoyable experience for everyone, where food becomes something fun and positive, not a battle.

Creating this kind of atmosphere doesn't have to be complicated! Simple little touches can completely change the vibe of mealtime. Try playing soft music in the background to set a calming mood, or add a bit of fun by decorating the table with a theme, such as a bright tablecloth or a vase of fresh flowers. These small details can make dinner feel special, almost like an event, and it might even spark your child's curiosity. It's all about building a space where they feel comfortable and excited to see what's next, making them more open to trying new foods without even realising it! As a child, I remember making 'name places' for my parents' dinner parties, so this can easily be incorporated into weekday family meals.

Of course, every family faces mealtime challenges. Tiredness and sibling rivalry can easily disrupt the peace. One solution is to involve each child in small tasks, like setting the table or serving food. This not only gives them a sense of responsibility but also channels their energy positively. If your child refuses to eat, try to manage it without conflict. Offer choices, such as deciding between two vegetables, which gives them a sense of control. Remember, it's okay if they don't eat everything. The goal is to keep the environment positive and pressure-free. Your patience and understanding can make all the difference.

Pia is usually pretty wiped out by mealtime, and sitting still isn't her strong suit! She's easily distracted and will often come up with reasons to leave the table, whether it's suddenly needing her toy or deciding she suddenly needs a wee halfway through. I know she's probably just trying to avoid eating her meal, so I'm working on being firmer with her about staying put during dinner. It's definitely a work in progress!

Remember, as a parent, you play a massive role in how mealtimes go. It's not just about what's on the plate—it's about the whole experience. By creating a positive, relaxed vibe, you're helping your child build a healthy relationship with food. Mealtimes can become something to look forward to, where trying new foods is just part of the fun and connection you share. It's about making those moments together enjoyable, not stressful!

Celebrating Small Wins: Incremental Changes

Picture this: your child takes their first bite of a vegetable they've always avoided. It's such a small moment, but it's a big win in the world of picky eating. Recognising these little victories is so important - it builds their confidence and motivates them to keep trying new foods. Even if it's just a tiny nibble or a quick lick, praising reinforces that positive behaviour and makes them proud of their effort. That encouragement can be the difference between a child who dreads mealtime and one who actually looks forward to it because they know their achievements will be noticed and celebrated.

Celebrating these wins doesn't need to be anything fancy. A simple food adventure chart where they earn a sticker for each new food they try can be a fun and motivating way for them to see their progress. You could also plan a special outing as a reward, such as a trip to the park or their favourite place. These experiences make trying new foods feel like an adventure, creating a positive cycle that keeps them excited to explore more!

Setting realistic goals is critical for getting your child to try new foods. Instead of bombarding them with too many changes at once, aim for just one new food a week. This way, they can explore variety within the foods they already know, making new things feel less daunting. It's all about finding that balance - challenging them enough but not so much that they feel overwhelmed. When the goals are small and manageable, they'll feel a sense of achievement, and that little boost in confidence will keep them excited to try more. It's a gradual process, but over time, it really does expand their palate!

I've seen this first-hand with Pia. During her pickiest era, she was the queen of beige foods; anything green was a hard pass. So, we set a goal of introducing one new green vegetable a week. We started small, literally, just one pea. Over time, we worked our way up to broccoli and even a bright green spinach pasta sauce (I never thought I'd see the day!). To keep it fun, she earned stickers for every bite and was so proud of her sticker chart. Slowly but surely, her plate went from bland to colourful. It didn't happen overnight, but the progress was amazing!

We added a little twist that worked wonders - letting Pia choose the new food herself. It became a weekly challenge where she picked something to try, and if she gave it a proper go, we'd plan a fun outing. More often than not, it meant an hour at her beloved (and my dreaded!) soft play. But honestly, if a few bites of broccoli earn me an hour of chaos in the ball pit, I'll take it!

It's all about celebrating those little victories. Every nibble is a win, building their confidence to try more. So, if you're dealing with a picky eater, too, don't stress. Keep it fun, be patient, and before you know it, they'll be trying new things. It's all about creating a low-pressure, positive vibe at the table—and maybe bribing them with soft play trips now and then!

As we wrap up this chapter, take a moment to reflect on the small wins you can celebrate with your child. These moments, while seemingly minor, are the building blocks of change. Creating a positive, encouraging environment will help promote healthier eating habits. With patience and persistence, you'll find that these incremental changes can lead to significant progress, setting the stage for the next chapter, where we'll explore engaging children in the kitchen.

What to Do Next:

1. Download and use the "Picky Eating Journal" PDF to track your child's food experiences and progress. It's included in the Bonus Pack at the front of the book.

2. Create a positive mealtime environment with regular timing, minimal distractions, and background music. Create a playlist and get everyone to add something.

3. Implement the no-pressure approach - offer new foods alongside established favourites without demands or repercussions if they are refused.

4. Set up a food adventure chart with stickers to celebrate trying new foods. Get your kid to add the stickers themselves and make a bit of a fuss about it!

5. Aim to introduce one new food per week, starting with small portions, and let your child choose what to try. Not everything will succeed but tdon't stress if it doesn't!

6. Use creative food presentation techniques to make meals more appealing. You can download our bonus pack that has a free PDF full of inspiration.

7. Involve children in meal preparation and table setting to increase their engagement. Rotate the tasks if you have more than one child every day to keep it fun.

8. Download and use the "Creative Meal Ideas" PDF, checking cupboards for ingredients and watching the recipe videos with your child. It's included in the Bonus Pack.

Chapter Three

Engaging Children in the Kitchen

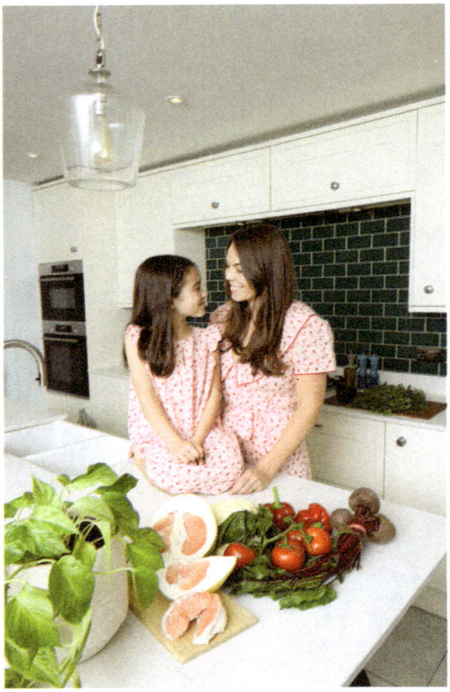
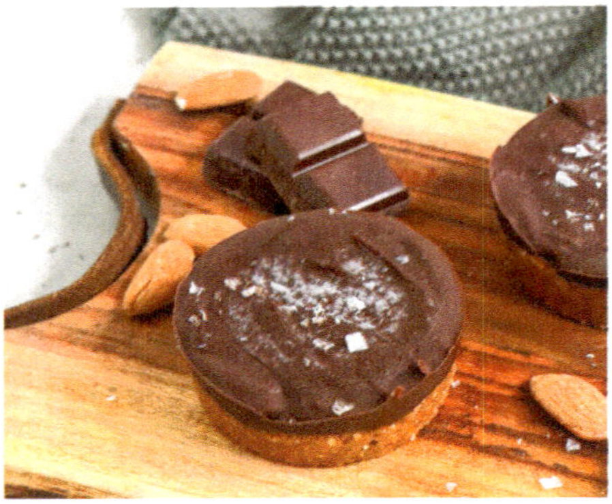
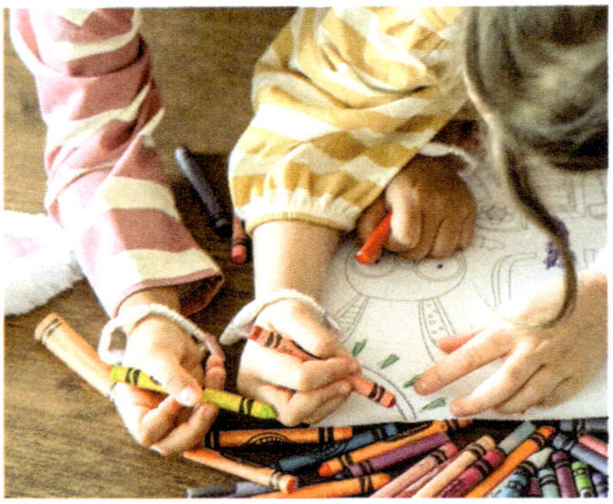
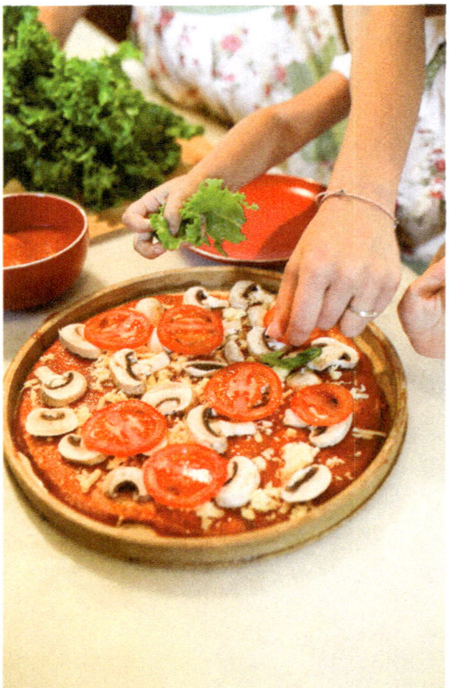

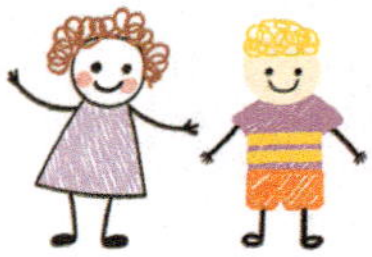

Engaging Children in the Kitchen

Picture your kitchen as a lively hub of creativity in your home - a place where mouthwatering smells fill the air, and your child stands proudly beside you, feeling more like a chef than just a spectator. This space can be a magical realm of learning and bonding where kids don't just eat but actively create! I know the thought of inviting your little ones into the kitchen can be a bit overwhelming, especially when you think about safety and keeping things organised. But transforming your kitchen into a child-friendly zone is totally doable, and it's all about encouraging exploration and independence.

The first step to making this vision a reality is to create a safe and accessible kitchen environment. It's essential that your child can get involved in cooking without putting themselves at risk. Adjustable stools can be a game-changer, letting your child reach the counter comfortably and safely. They get a better view of the action and gain confidence as they stand tall, ready to tackle whatever task you throw their way. We have been using the Stokke Trip Trapp for years, and you can adjust it with age. It doubles up as a brilliant stool for mini sous-chefs! Then there are utensils; investing in child-safe tools is a smart move. Look for items with nonslip grips or ergonomic handles that fit perfectly in those tiny hands. This way, your child can easily chop, stir, and mix, making the whole experience enjoyable for both of you!

I have created a list of my favourite, kid-friendly kitchen utensils for you on my Amazon shopfront, so feel free to take a look by clicking on the link or scanning the QR code.

Organising the kitchen

Organising your kitchen to encourage young cooks is another vital aspect. Consider designating a low cabinet specifically for your child's tools and ingredients. This gives them easy access and instils a sense of ownership and responsibility. You might also label containers with pictures, making it easier for them to identify ingredients. This simple step can turn a chaotic kitchen into a space where your child can independently gather what they need, fostering confidence and a sense of independence. Such organisation can make cooking less intimidating and more inviting, transforming your child from a passive observer into an active participant.

Involving your child in organising the kitchen can be incredibly beneficial. Assign them specific tasks like sorting utensils or arranging ingredients. Not only does this help them feel more connected to the space, but it also teaches them responsibility and the importance of maintaining order. Creating a weekly schedule for restocking ingredients can be another valuable lesson. By involving your child in checking pantry items and making shopping lists, you encourage them to take ownership of their contributions to family meals. These activities can help build essential life skills that extend beyond the kitchen, fostering a sense of accomplishment and pride.

Personalising the kitchen space can make it even more inviting for your child. Displaying their artwork or recipe creations on the fridge or walls can instil a sense of pride and belonging. They'll see the kitchen as a place where their contributions are valued and celebrated. Consider using colourful mats and aprons to add a touch of fun and personalisation. These simple additions can make the kitchen feel like their domain, a place where they are empowered to experiment and learn. Personal touches can inspire creativity and make your child more eager to spend time cooking with you, turning routine meals into cherished family experiences.

CLEMMIE'S Tip

Pia's Pizza Recipe

I just had to include Pia's favourite Pizza Recipe, just for the wonderful hand written instructions! I love the "Wear a chef's hat!"

Watch use make these in the video or scan the QR code

Can we talk about flour for a minute? Because this really makes all the difference

Instrutions on how too make Marguerita

You will need:

- Dough
- Pan
- Tomato saes
- Spoon
- cheese
- Flour
- oven
- box

Firsty wash your hands.
Second, Put on apron and wear a chef hat.
Third) get a pan with dough.
Fourth, thikon the edge.
Fifth, spred the Tomato saes on the dough.
Sixth Put the cheese
seventh Put it in the oven(371°c) For four minutes to cook.
Eight) take it out and put it in a box.
Finally Injoy eting your pissa.

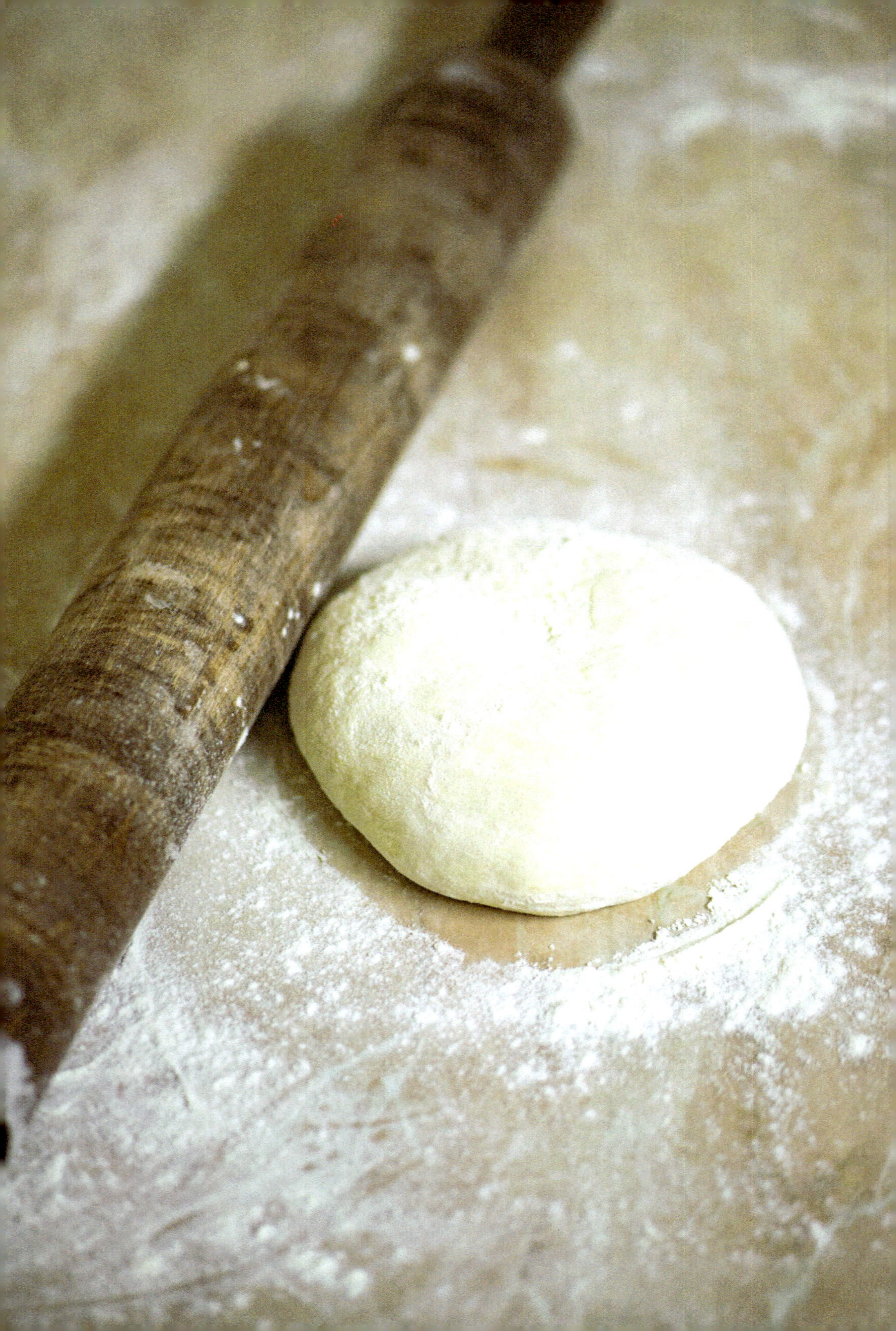

PIA'S PIZZA

Prep: 20 Mins Prove: 60 mins

The easier to read version of Pia's Margherita Pizza recipe!

Makes 6 small pizzas

1kg strong white bread flour or Tipo '00' flour, (or 800g strong white bread flour or Tipo '00' flour, **plus** 200g finely ground semolina flour)

1 teaspoon fine sea salt

2 x 7g sachets of dried yeast

1 tablespoon golden caster sugar

4 tablespoons extra virgin olive oil

Toppings: Tomato Sauce, Passatta, Mozarella, Pepporoni. Veggies etc

Instructions

Wash your hands and put on an Apron and Chef's hat!

Sieve the flour/s and salt on to a clean work surface and make a well in the middle.

In a jug, mix the yeast, sugar and oil into 650ml of lukewarm water and leave for a few minutes, then pour into the well.

Using a fork, bring the flour in gradually from the sides and swirl it into the liquid. until it all starts to come together, Knead until you have a smooth, springy dough.

Place the ball of dough in a large flour-dusted bowl and flour the top of it. Cover the bowl with a damp cloth and place in a warm room for about an hour until the dough has doubled in size (Proving)

Now remove the dough to a flour-dusted surface and knead it around a bit to push the air out with your hands – this is called knocking back the dough. You can either use it immediately, or keep it, wrapped in clingfilm, in the fridge (or freezer) until required.

If using straight away, divide the dough up into as many little balls as you want to make pizzas – this amount of dough is enough to make about six to eight medium pizzas.

CLEMMIE'S Tip

Try to use the Italian Tipo '00' flour - it's this super-fine flour that makes your dough feel like silk between good pizza and "oh my goodness, this is amazing" pizza! I learned this after several attempts where even Pia's stuffed animals weren't impressed. Then I discovered Italian Tipo '00' flour - it's this super-fine flour that makes your dough feel like silk and you can usually find it in Italian food shops or bigger supermarkets. If you can't get the Italian stuff, don't panic! Just look for strong white bread flour with high gluten content, and try mixing in a bit of semolina flour for gorgeous color and flavor.

Simple Recipes for Little Chefs

Picture this: your child, apron on and beaming with pride, stands beside you, ready to whip up something delicious they can call their own. Simple, fun recipes can turn them from little helpers into culinary adventurers. Start with some peanut butter cups—perfect for those eager little hands to mix the ingredients together. They'll love the process and the result: a tasty snack they created all by themselves!

Peanut Butter Cups

CLEMMIE'S Tip

Quick and easy peanut butter cups - perfect little afternoon treat - keep them in the freezer for a quick, nutritious snack!

Watch us make these in the video or scan the QR code.

Another easy winner is fruit and yoghurt parfaits, where they can layer their favourite fruits and granola. Not only will this fill their tummies, but it'll also warm their hearts with a sense of pride and accomplishment.

Cooking isn't just about what comes out of the oven; it's a learning experience. Each recipe serves as a sneaky little lesson. Measuring ingredients teaches your child about fractions and volume, especially when they see how different amounts affect the mix - maths without the textbook, and it's delicious! And mixing? It might seem simple, but it helps develop those fine motor skills. When they're manoeuvring a spoon through thick batter or a creamy mixture, they're building coordination and strength. These activities aren't just fun; they're essential life skills in the making.

To make these lessons even more engaging, create illustrated recipe cards with step-by-step instructions and pictures. These visual aids can help guide your child through the process. If you feel tech-savvy, add video tutorials that are accessible via QR codes for a little extra interaction. Watching a quick clip of a chef - maybe even a child chef, preparing the same recipe can spark their interest and help them feel connected to the process. These tools transform cooking into an adventure where your child learns by seeing and doing - a multi-sensory experience that

Interactive Element: Kid-Friendly Kitchen Checklist

Make it a fun activity by creating a checklist with your child to ensure their kitchen space is organised and safe. You can include questions like "Is the stool stable?" or "Gather my cooking tools from the cabinet." This will make preparing for each cooking session an enjoyable and educational experience while reinforcing the importance of safety and organisation.

By making the kitchen a welcoming and accessible space, you can create countless bonding opportunities while teaching your child valuable skills. It's all about creating an environment that invites exploration and learning, where your child feels safe and inspired to dive into meal prep and become an integral part of the cooking adventure!

You can either click to download my example checklist which is included in our Bonus Pack or scan the QR code.

captures their imagination.

But don't stop there! Encourage your child to get creative and experiment. Maybe they want to toss in a sprinkle of cinnamon to their energy bites or swap strawberries for bananas in their parfait. Let them go wild! This kind of experimentation nurtures their creativity and builds confidence in the kitchen. It teaches them that recipes are guidelines, not strict rules. When they add their favourite toppings to a homemade pizza or mix different fruits into a smoothie, they're not just cooking; they're innovating. That freedom to explore can lead to delightful surprises and a greater sense of ownership over their culinary creations.

Cooking with your child can be one of the most rewarding experiences ever. It's a chance to bond, teach, and learn together. As they master these simple recipes, they'll build confidence and independence, turning the kitchen into a playground of flavours and textures. So grab those aprons, gather your ingredients, and let the culinary adventures begin!

Fun with Food: Creative Cooking Activities

Turning cooking into a playful activity often sparks Pia's creativity and curiosity. One of our favourite ways to do this is by making 'rainbow' fruit kebabs. Pia loves selecting her favourite fruits, threading them onto the skewers, and creating her own colourful masterpiece. This fun activity encourages her to explore new flavours and textures, making healthy eating exciting and enjoyable.

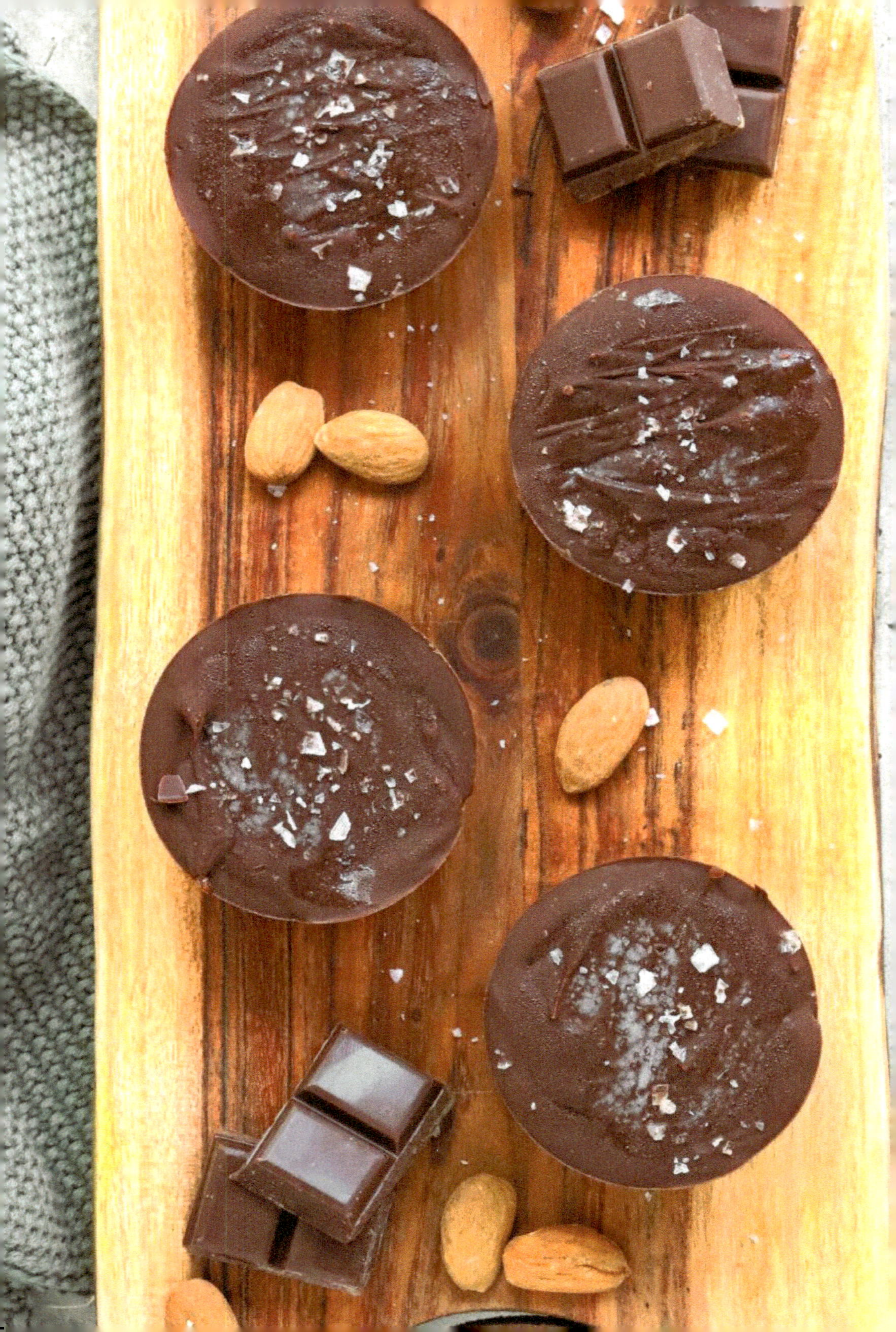

PEANUT BUTTER CUPS

Prep: 40 Mins

Quick and easy peanut butter cups - perfect little afternoon treat - keep them in the freezer for a quick, nutritious snack!

Serves 6

1 cup Medjool dates, pitted

1 cup rolled oats

1 cup walnuts

1/4 cup flax seeds, ground

1 teaspoon vanilla extract

1/2 teaspoon cinnamon, ground

Pinch of salt

Vegan dark chocolate, melted (for drizzling)

Water, if needed

Instructions

Place the coconut oil and chocolate chips into a small pot and melt over low heat.

Remove from the heat before the chocolate chips have fully melted.

Meanwhile, mix together the almond milk, peanut butter, protein powder and vanilla extract.

Press the peanut butter mixture into mini silicone muffin moulds.

Make sure to press down hard so that the mixture sticks together.

Pour the melted chocolate over the top, dividing the chocolate equally between each peanut butter cup.

Place into the freezer to set.

CLEMMIE'S Tip

I would recommend that you use sustainable Peanut Butter that Palm oil free.

Our favourite is Pippin Nut and there is a 15% discount code in our Supplier section on

They also do an awesome Almond Nut butter which is slightly higher in Protein.

We also enjoy making sandwiches using cookie cutters to create fun shapes (see my Amazon shop!). The delight on Pia's face when her usual sandwich becomes a star or a dinosaur is priceless. I love giving her the freedom to choose the shapes while I guide her as she presses down on the bread. This turns her lunches into a creative experience, allowing her to feel ownership over her meal. It even leads to conversations about shapes and geometry, sneaking in some learning while we have fun!

Themed Cooking Days

Themed cooking days are a hit in our household, turning dinner into a festive occasion. For example, on Taco Tuesday, we create a DIY toppings bar filled with salsa, guacamole, cheese, and beans, allowing Pia to take on the role of chef as she assembles her tacos. This interactive experience makes mealtime fun and encourages her to explore various flavour combinations at her own pace. The possibilities are endless! You might consider hosting International Nights, diving into a different country's cuisine each week. Whether indulging in Italian pasta or an Indian curry, these themed dinners can help broaden your child's palate and enhance their cultural awareness.

To make cooking even more special by turning each meal into a part of a larger story. I remember one evening when we crafted mini-pizzas while I shared a little video on how pizza was invented - Pia was utterly captivated! This connection to the history and culture behind the food enriches her appreciation for what we're creating together. It reminds me of my own travels when I was younger, where discovering new foods was always tied to the stories of the places I visited. By incorporating this element into our cooking, I'm not just teaching her how to make meals; I'm helping her appreciate the cultures and traditions that food represents, which is so important, particularly as she is half South American!

With each activity, Pia is learning about food and hopefully developing a love for the process. These playful cooking experiences create lasting memories and instil a lifelong appreciation for healthy eating and cooking.

Building Confidence: Kids as Sous Chefs

Having Pia in the kitchen with me allows her to build confidence and learn essential skills. We start with simple tasks, like washing fruits and vegetables, which provides a tactile experience that's both educational and engaging. As she becomes more comfortable, I introduce her to slightly more complex duties, such as tearing lettuce for salads or arranging ingredients on a cutting board. Each time she completes a task, her self-esteem grows, reinforcing her role as a valuable contributor to our family meals.

Positive feedback plays a huge role in this process. When I offer encouragement and praise, I can see how valued Pia feels, motivating her to keep learning. I focus on her efforts rather than just the results. For example, if she chops carrots and some pieces are uneven, I celebrate the fact that she tried and learned from the experience. This helps cultivate a growth mindset, where she understands that skills improve with practice. As her confidence builds, she becomes eager to tackle more challenging tasks, like stirring a simmering pot or cracking an egg.

I believe in gradually increasing responsibilities in the kitchen. We start with familiar tasks like setting the table or mixing ingredients. Once she's comfortable, I guide her in using a safe, child-friendly knife to chop soft vegetables. This step-by-step approach builds her culinary skills and a sense of pride and ownership. Before long, she might even feel confident enough to prepare a simple dish all on her own!

Working together in the kitchen also strengthens our bond. Planning a meal together allows us to share ideas and preferences, encouraging teamwork. I like to assign roles based on each person's strengths and interests - maybe Pia will wash the veggies while I measure the ingredients. This encourages communication and cooperation, bringing us closer as we work towards a common goal. These experiences not only enhance our culinary skills but also deepen our connections and create lasting memories. Most of our childhood memories come from everyday experiences rather than big occasions.

I vividly remember my dad teaching my sister and me how to make a variety of sauces: cheese sauce, chocolate sauce, barbecue sauce, gravy, and dressings. He truly was the king of sauces! Before long, my sister and I were whipping them up on our own, and that newfound confidence transformed cooking into a passion of mine. I still make these sauces today, and mastering these basic flavour combinations is such a valuable skill.

If you have multiple children, consider how they can collaborate to create a signature dish for a family dinner. They can brainstorm ideas, experiment with flavours, and craft a meal that becomes a family favourite. These experiences not only empower kids in the kitchen but also lead to remarkable achievements and foster a lifelong love for cooking.

As you getting kids more involved in the kitchen, remember that confidence and skills develop with each task they tackle. By encouraging independence and teamwork, we're helping shape future chefs who will carry these important lessons throughout their lives. Next, we'll explore how to handle dietary restrictions.

What to do Next

1. Create a child-friendly kitchen environment with safe utensils, adjustable stools, and a designated low cabinet for their tools and workspace.

2. Personalise their kitchen space with artwork and labelled containers using pictures drawn by your kids or to inspire them about a task or new vegetable

3. Make a Kid-Friendly Kitchen Checklist, including reviewing recommended kitchen utensils for small hands. Some great suppliers are listed in Chapter 14.

4. Start with basic tasks like washing produce, then gradually teach new skills such as using child-friendly knives, peeling fruit or how to measure quantities.

5. Create illustrated recipe cards and watch tutorial videos together for guidance. Build up a mini-library of their favourite dishes and get them to use them and rate them.

6. Plan engaging activities like "rainbow" fruit kebabs and themed cooking days (e.g., Taco Tuesday) to help introduce new flavours and increase their curiosity.

7. Check cupboards and create shopping lists for starter recipes (no-bake energy bites, fruit and yoghurt parfaits) so that you always have something fun in stock.

8. Assign age-appropriate kitchen roles to family members based on their interests and abilities. You can rotate them through different roles to ensure fairness too!

Chapter Four

Dealing with Dietary Restrictions

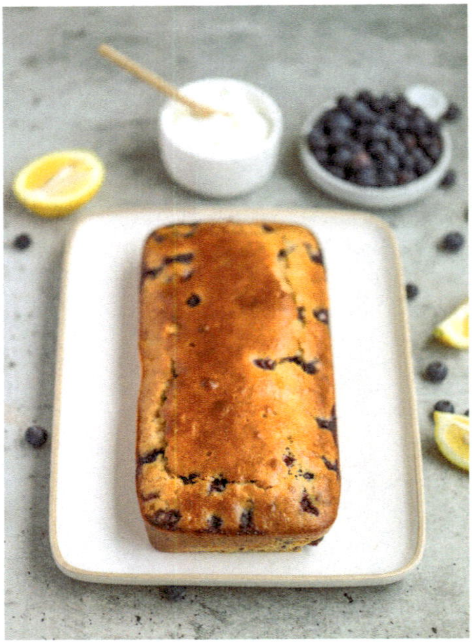

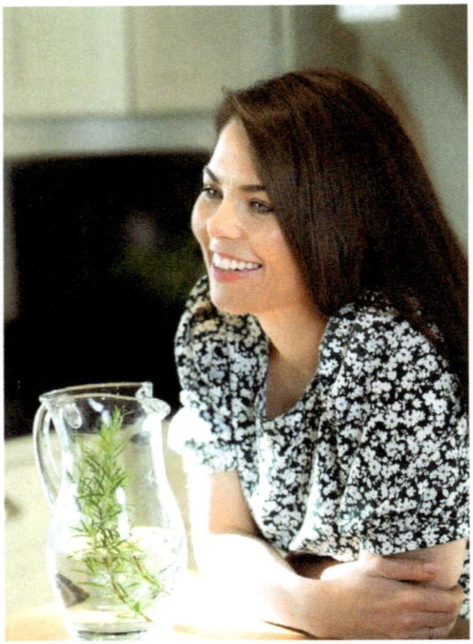

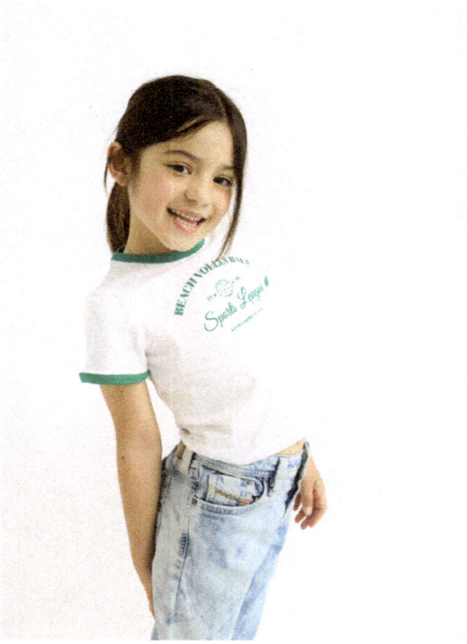

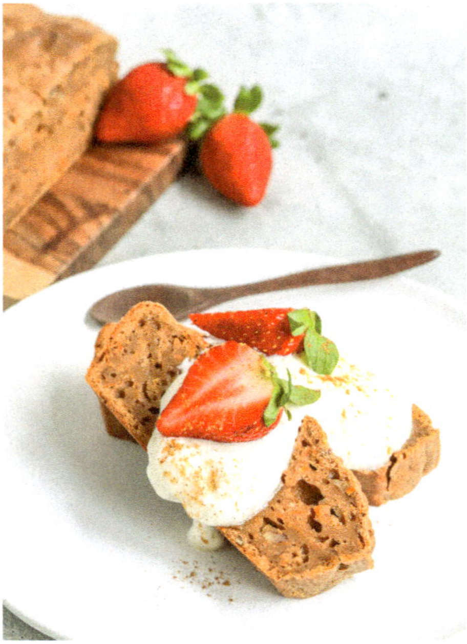

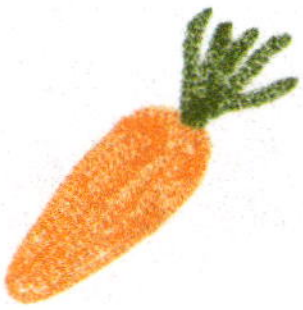

Dealing with Dietary Restrictions

Every year, when I'm prepping for Pia's birthday party, the house buzzes with excitement. The obligatory 'happy birthday' banner is up, balloons float around, and the smell of freshly baked cupcakes fills the air - pure nostalgia! However, as I make her favourite treats, there's always that little flicker of worry - what if one of her friends has a food allergy? How do I make sure every child is safe and still has the best time? Navigating dietary restrictions feels like walking a tightrope, trying to balance safety with fun. But understanding common allergies and intolerances has become essential when creating a party where every child feels included, safe, and ready to enjoy the day - so much to think about!

Around 1 in 50 children in the UK and about 1 in 40 in the USA are affected by peanut allergies, making it one of the most common food allergies among kids. Nut allergies are also on the rise, with studies showing that the number of children with peanut allergies has tripled in recent decades.

CLEMMIE'S Tip

A really good fact sheet is available from Alllergyuk, but a simple Google search will provide up to date statistics, resources and organisations that can help you to understand the facts better and create some coping mechanisms.

Let's clear up the difference between allergies and intolerances because it's so easy to confuse them, but they impact the body in entirely different ways. Allergies involve the immune system going into overdrive. It's like your child's body mistaking a perfectly harmless peanut for something dangerous, triggering alarms that can lead to hives, swelling, or, in extreme cases, anaphylaxis – a severe reaction that needs urgent medical attention. Intolerances, however, tend to be gentler on the body and are more about digestion. For example, a child with lactose intolerance might feel uncomfortable or have an upset stomach after milk, but it's not life-threatening. It can usually be managed with some simple dietary adjustments.

Understanding the most common food allergens is a huge step in managing them day-to-day. According to the Centres for Disease Control and Prevention (CDC), eight foods are responsible for the majority of severe allergic reactions: milk, eggs, peanuts, tree nuts, soy, wheat, fish, and shellfish. These allergens can sneak into foods where you'd least expect them, so becoming a label-reading pro is essential. For example, soy could hide in your child's favourite snack, and tree nuts might pop up in sauces. Recognising allergic reaction symptoms such as hives or trouble breathing is essential for acting fast and preventing severe consequences. Over 40% of children with food allergies in the U.S. have had to visit emergency rooms, so being prepared and vigilant is vital.

The reasons behind food allergies in children are a bit of a puzzle, influenced by genetics and the environment. If you or your partner have allergies, there's a higher chance your child will be more susceptible, too. But it's not just down to genetics—environmental factors also come into play. For instance, introducing allergens such as peanuts early on has been shown to lower the risk of allergies developing.

I was so adamant that Pia wasn't going to have a nut allergy that I started spoon-feeding her nut butter when she was a baby! I'd heard about the benefits of early exposure, and I was determined she wouldn't have any issues. Fast forward, and now we're both total nut butter addicts - whether it's on toast, in smoothies, or just straight out of the jar! Early choices can make such a difference. Here in the UK, food allergies are on the rise, with around 5-8% of children affected, so staying informed is more important than ever.

Spotting and managing food allergies early on is so important for your child's safety and your peace of mind. If you think your child might have an allergy, it's worth getting professional advice immediately. Allergy testing can give you clarity and help you figure out exactly what the triggers are. Once you know, it's all about teamwork—between you, your child, and healthcare professionals. Creating an allergy action plan is a must, laying out precisely what to do if your child is exposed, whether that's giving them antihistamines or using an EpiPen in severe cases. It's your go-to guide for handling any emergency quickly and calmly.

As a nutritionist, I'm here to help, too! Feel free to reach out if you're unsure which tests to take or have received results and need support managing allergies through diet. I can guide you through the process and offer personalised advice to keep your child safe and well.

Interactive Element: Allergy Action Plan Template

Create a personalised allergy action plan that's super clear. We've included a template in our Bonus Pack - the QR code is at the front of the book. Ensure it includes easy-to-follow instructions for spotting symptoms and when to give emergency meds. Share it with anyone who cares for your child, including caregivers and schools, so everyone is on the same page and ready to act.

Managing food allergies can sometimes feel overwhelming, but with the proper knowledge and a bit of planning, it becomes much more manageable. Understanding the difference between allergies and intolerances, recognising the signs, and having a solid action plan in place are key. With these tools, you can confidently keep your child safe while they still enjoy all the fun and excitement life has to offer.

Allergy-Friendly Substitutions and Swaps

It's birthday cake time, and you suddenly remember that one of the kids can't have eggs. Cue the panic for a second! But then I remind myself of all the great substitutes out there. Navigating food allergies doesn't mean sacrificing taste or nutrition - thankfully, there are plenty of delicious options!

When Pia was younger, I remember baking with one of her friends. Just as we were about to crack the eggs, I realised her friend couldn't have them. Instead of throwing in the towel, I recalled a baking video I'd watched that suggested using applesauce as a substitute. Luckily, I had some in the cupboard! It worked perfectly, and the cake turned out as moist and delicious as ever. It's funny how those moments can spark our creativity in the kitchen!

Dairy is another common allergen, but I've discovered that oat, almond, and coconut milk are excellent alternatives. These options mimic the creaminess of cow's milk and are frequently fortified with essential nutrients like calcium and vitamin D, ensuring the little ones get everything they need.

I personally love using Plenish milks because they're free from unnecessary additives. Just a tip: it's best to avoid nut milks that contain seed oils, as they can be tough on digestion. Highly processed seed oils often contain omega-6 fatty acids, which can promote inflammation when consumed in excess. For those with sensitive digestive systems, these oils can lead to bloating, gas, or other gastrointestinal discomfort. So, opting for nut milks without these added oils can be a gentler choice for digestion and little tummies!

These small swaps can help maintain nutritional value without compromising on taste. For example, using a flaxseed meal mixed with water as an egg replacer is a game changer. Imagine whipping up vegan pancakes with banana and oat milk—the banana acts as a binder and sweetener, while the oat milk keeps them fluffy.

Of course, cross-contamination is a big concern when making allergy-friendly meals. I always use separate utensils and cutting boards to keep allergens from sneaking into safe foods. It might seem like an extra step, but it's so important! Educating family members about allergy safety protocols also goes a long way. Everyone must be on the same page about which foods are safe and how to handle them properly. This teamwork makes things so much easier and creates a safer kitchen environment for everyone.

Cooking with substitutes is all about creativity and adaptability. Whether you're baking a cake or preparing a family dinner, these swaps allow you to cater to everyone's needs without feeling overwhelmed. With some knowledge and the right ingredients, you can whip up delicious, allergy-friendly dishes that are just as nourishing as they are tasty.

Food allergies can be managed with the proper knowledge and planning. Get creative with substitutions, such as using applesauce instead of eggs or fortified plant-based milks instead of cow's milk. Always prioritise safety by preventing cross-contamination and educating everyone involved in food prep. If you're uncertain about what to do or need support, don't hesitate to reach out! Together, we can ensure your family safely enjoys all the deliciousness life has to offer!

Building a Diverse and Safe Pantry

Imagine your cupboards/pantry as a treasure trove brimming with ingredients ready to fuel your family's meals. Stocking it thoughtfully sets the stage for culinary success, especially when food allergies are a concern. Your first line of defence? Choosing certified allergen-free products. These items undergo rigorous testing to ensure they're free from traces of common allergens. Always look for labels that clearly indicate they're free from the specific allergens you're avoiding. This careful selection acts as a safety net, offering peace of mind as you prepare meals for your loved ones.

Once your cupboards are well-stocked, clear labelling becomes essential, especially when you're in a rush to make dinner, only to grab the wrong pasta. This is where labels come to the rescue! They prevent mix-ups and help maintain an allergy-safe zone in your kitchen.

Consider using colour-coded labels or bold markers to make it easy for anyone - whether it's you, your partner, or a babysitter to navigate your kitchen without worry. This small step can make a big difference in ensuring everyone's safety and keeping your cooking stress-free!

CLEMMIE'S Tip

It's actually quite a therapeutic activity if you love re-organising stuff as much as I do! I love using this label machine which you can get from my Amazon shop.

Variety is the spice of life, as they say, and it's no different when creating an allergy-friendly pantry. Incorporating diverse ingredient options keeps meals interesting and balanced. Grains such as quinoa, millet, and amaranth are fantastic gluten-free options. They're not just substitutes; they're nutrition powerhouses that offer unique flavours and textures to your meals. Quinoa, for instance, is rich in protein and fibre, making it a perfect 'complete protein' for salads or as a side dish. Millet and amaranth can be cooked into porridge or added to soups for an extra nutritional punch. Alternative protein sources, such as lentils and chickpeas, are also wonderful. They're versatile, nourishing, and can be used in a myriad of dishes - think lentil stews or chickpea salads. These ingredients ensure your meals are safe and packed with nutrients and flavour.

Planning meals around pantry staples can make your life easier and meals more predictable. Start by creating a weekly meal plan that revolves around what you already have. This not only saves you time but also reduces food waste. Identify the staples you use most often (rice, beans, or canned tomatoes, for example) and build your meals around them. Rotating these staple recipes ensures variety and keeps everyone from getting bored. Maybe Monday is for a hearty quinoa salad, while Tuesday features a comforting chickpea curry. By setting a routine, you streamline your shopping trips and avoid the last-minute scramble for missing ingredients!

If you're super organised (which, to be honest, is a work in progress for me!), doing monthly pantry audits is a fantastic way to keep your kitchen safe and efficient. It's simple: go through your pantry, check for expired products, and toss them out to avoid accidental use. This keeps your space tidy and ensures everything you have is fresh and safe to eat.

When it comes to allergen-free products, it's crucial to ensure they stay uncontaminated. Always check the packaging for any signs of damage that might introduce allergens. This little routine keeps your pantry organised and reinforces the habit of being mindful about what you're feeding your family. It may seem like a small task, but the benefits are enormous—ensuring every meal you prepare is as safe and nutritious as possible! Plus, it's a great excuse to rediscover some of those hidden gems in the back of the cupboard.

Your pantry isn't just a place to stash ingredients; it's the beating heart of your kitchen! By selecting safe products, mixing up your ingredients, planning ahead, and doing regular audits, you're crafting an environment that promotes safety and creativity. It's all about striking that perfect balance between being cautious and exploring new flavours while ensuring your family's dietary needs are met with love and attention. Think of it as your culinary playground, where every meal is a chance to create something delicious and safe for everyone at the table!

Communicating Allergies to Caregivers and Schools

You're sending your child off to school or a playdate, hoping they'll have a fun and carefree day. But when food allergies are involved, that hope quickly turns into a necessity. It's so important to share clear and detailed allergy information with caregivers and schools—think of it as sharing the vital details about your child's health. This means putting together written instructions that highlight specific allergens to avoid, the symptoms of an allergic reaction, and emergency contacts to call if needed. It's all about creating a safety net that extends beyond your watchful eye to include teachers, babysitters, and anyone else who might be responsible for your little one. They need to know exactly what to do and who to contact if something goes awry. By sharing this info upfront, you help ensure your child can enjoy their time away from home with minimal risk.

Having an allergy action plan is a game-changer! Think of it as a step-by-step guide for handling any allergic reactions that might pop up. This plan should detail how to spot symptoms, how to use medications like EpiPens, and the exact steps to take in an emergency. Providing templates for these plans can make everything smoother for everyone involved. These documents serve as a clear roadmap, reducing panic and confusion during stressful moments. You can tailor these templates to fit your child's unique needs, ensuring all caregivers know what to do and feel equipped to act quickly. This preparation isn't just about managing emergencies; it's about giving you peace of mind, knowing you've done everything possible to keep your child safe.

Understanding your child's legal rights is another essential layer of protection. Schools and daycares have a responsibility to accommodate these needs, often through 504 Plans. These legally binding agreements outline how schools will ensure your child's safety and access to education. Knowing your child's rights empowers you to advocate for necessary accommodations, like allergen-free zones or tailored lunch plans. It's all about creating a safe space where your child can learn and thrive without the constant worry of exposure to allergens. Legal protections are there for a reason, so don't hesitate to leverage them to your advantage.

Empowering your child to communicate their needs is just as crucial. Teaching them to recognise their allergies and express them to others is a valuable life skill. Encourage them to speak up in social settings, whether at school or a friend's house. Role-playing can be a great way to prepare them for real-life situations, helping them practice what to say if they're offered food that might contain allergens. This self-advocacy boosts their confidence and reinforces the importance of taking their allergies seriously. It's all about equipping them with the knowledge and courage to protect themselves, even when you're not around.

As you learn to cope with your child's allergies, remember that communication is critical. Creating a network of informed and prepared individuals is vital for supporting your child's health and well-being. With clear communication, detailed plans, and empowered children, you can ensure your child's world is as safe and inclusive as possible.

What to do Next

- Create a personalised Allergy Action Plan template for your child, including emergency contacts and specific symptoms and share it with others such as teachers.
- Create a clear labelling system for your pantry with colour-coded markers for allergen-free foods and potential allergens. Use a labelling machine to provide consistency.
- Set up an allergen-free zone in your kitchen with separate utensils and cutting boards to prevent cross-contamination. You can label the boards for the different food types
- Stock your pantry with certified allergen-free alternatives and safe substitutes (like applesauce for eggs, plant-based milks) and add them to your shopping list as a recurring item
- Practice role-playing scenarios with your child to help them communicate their allergies confidently. Focus on Physical symptoms such as breathing, itching a or aches.
- Write detailed allergy information sheets for caregivers, schools, and family members. Make sure you keep them up to date and reissue them termly.
- Review and familiarise yourself with symptoms of common allergies and proper use of emergency medications. Makes sure you have these on hand.

Join local allergy support groups or online communities for ongoing advice and recipe ideas. You can also join our Facebook group where there is a lively discussion.

Chapter Five

Gut Health for Kids

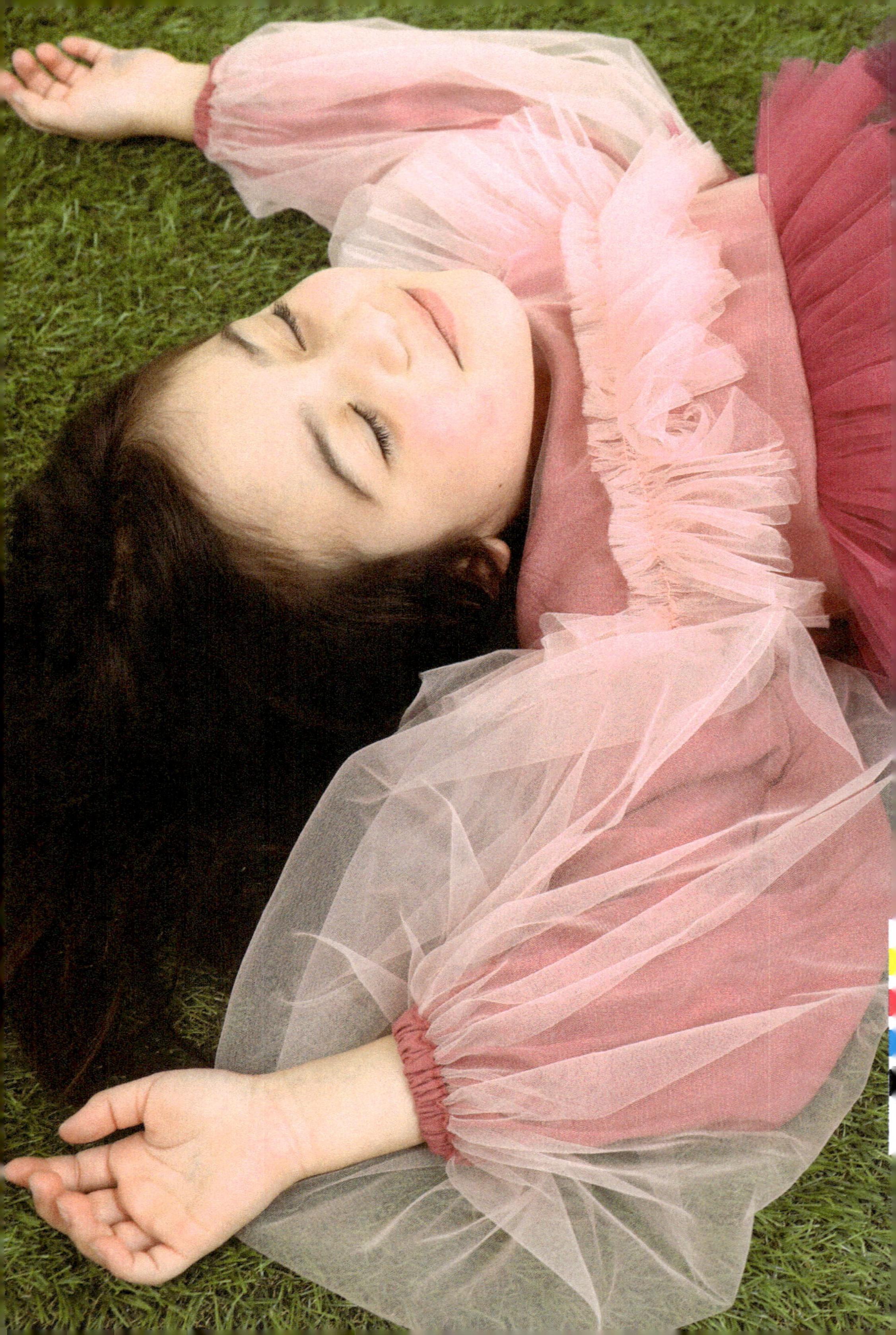

Gut Health for Kids

It's such a joy to see your child playing happily, full of energy and in high spirits. But behind the scenes, there's an unsung hero at work—their gut microbiome, or as I like to call it with Pia, the 'gut garden.' This thriving ecosystem of bacteria, viruses, and fungi in their intestines plays a crucial role in their overall health and well-being. By understanding the gut microbiome, you're unlocking the key to strengthening your child's immune system and laying the foundation for lifelong health.

What is a Microbiome

So, what exactly is this microbiome, and why does it matter so much? Let's dive into this fascinating inner world and explore how we can explain it to our kids!

The gut microbiome is made up of trillions of tiny microorganisms that live in our digestive tracts. Think of them as little superheroes, each with their own unique job! Some help break down the food we eat, while others produce vitamins that keep us strong. Many are vital for a healthy immune system. These microorganisms aren't just hanging out; they actively interact with your child's body, influencing everything from digestion to how well they fight off colds and infections.

To help your kids understand this concept, here are some fun ideas:

CLEMMIE'S Tip

Storytelling: Create a story about the "Superhero Microbes" who live in our bellies and protect us from harmful germs. You could give them names and explain their superpowers, like "Captain Fibre" for the microbes that help digest food or "Vitamin Squad" for those that create essential vitamins to keep us well.

CLEMMIE'S Tip

Visuals: Use colourful diagrams or videos to show what the gut looks like and how these microorganisms work together. You can find kid-friendly animations online that illustrate how the gut microbiome supports health.

CLEMMIE'S Tip

Hands-On Activities: Consider simple experiments, like growing bean sprouts or observing how different foods change the texture or taste of dishes. This can help children see how various foods nourish our gut heroes.

CLEMMIE'S Tip

Food Exploration: Involve your kids in cooking and meal prep. Talk about how certain foods, such as yoghurt, sauerkraut, and fruits, feed the good microbes and help them stay strong. You could even have a "microbe-friendly meal" night where you focus on including these foods.

CLEMMIE'S Tip

Questions and Curiosity: Let's inspire them to ask questions! If they're curious about why fruits and vegetables are so important, share how these foods fuel their little gut superheroes and keep them healthy and strong. Kids are naturally curious and often smarter than we give them credit for! It's such a gift to equip them with the knowledge to care for their guts from a young age, setting them up for a lifetime of optimal health!

By using engaging storytelling, visuals, hands-on activities, and discussions, we can make the concept of the gut microbiome relatable and fun for our children!

Microbiome Development

But how does this microbiome develop, especially in children? From the moment they enter the world, a child's gut microbiome begins its journey. The first 1,000 days are particularly critical for this development, with the foundation laid by factors like the mode of delivery, breastfeeding, and early diet. For example, children born via vaginal delivery typically have access to beneficial maternal bacteria, which can jumpstart a diverse microbiome. Breastfeeding also plays a vital role, introducing beneficial bacteria like Bifidobacterium species essential for immune system maturation.

Mums - I don't want you to start panicking if you didn't give birth naturally or breastfeed - it's okay! You can still have a very happy, healthy baby. There are many ways to support your child's microbiome, such as providing a varied and balanced diet rich in fibre and probiotics as they grow. These initial exposures play a crucial role in shaping their gut environment and influencing their health outcomes throughout life, regardless of how they started their journey.

As children grow, their microbiome evolves and adapts to their changing diets and environments. Introducing a wide range of foods - especially fruits, vegetables, and whole grains, helps cultivate a diverse microbial community. This diversity is vital because it helps prevent inflammatory and autoimmune disorders and supports neurological development.

Did you know that a healthy microbiome can even influence mood and behaviour? Studies now suggest that gut bacteria communicate with our brains, potentially affecting mental health and cognitive function. We now know that most of our happy hormone 'serotonin' (over 95%) is produced in the gut! So, a thriving microbiome isn't just about dodging illness - it's about building resilience and fostering optimal growth in all areas of life!

I know nurturing the gut microbiome can feel overwhelming to many parents, but it comes down to a few simple, consistent habits. Consider including a variety of whole foods in their meals and creating a calm, stress-free environment. When you support your child's microbiome, you're not just tackling short-term health issues but building a solid foundation for their future. This support can help them thrive in ways that go way beyond gut health!

Interactive Element: Microbiome Mood Journal

Create a "Microbiome Mood Journal" with your child. Track their meals and note any changes in mood or energy. Reflect on how different foods might impact their well-being. This can be a fun way to help them understand the connection between diet and health.

Factors Affecting Gut Health

Imagine your child enjoying a plate full of colourful fruits and vegetables while their gut is hard at work digesting all those nutrients. It may seem simple, but their diet plays a significant role in shaping their gut microbiome—or, as I like to call it with Pia, the 'gut garden.' The foods they eat either help their gut garden flourish or cause it to wilt.

High-fibre foods such as whole grains, fruits, and vegetables are like water and

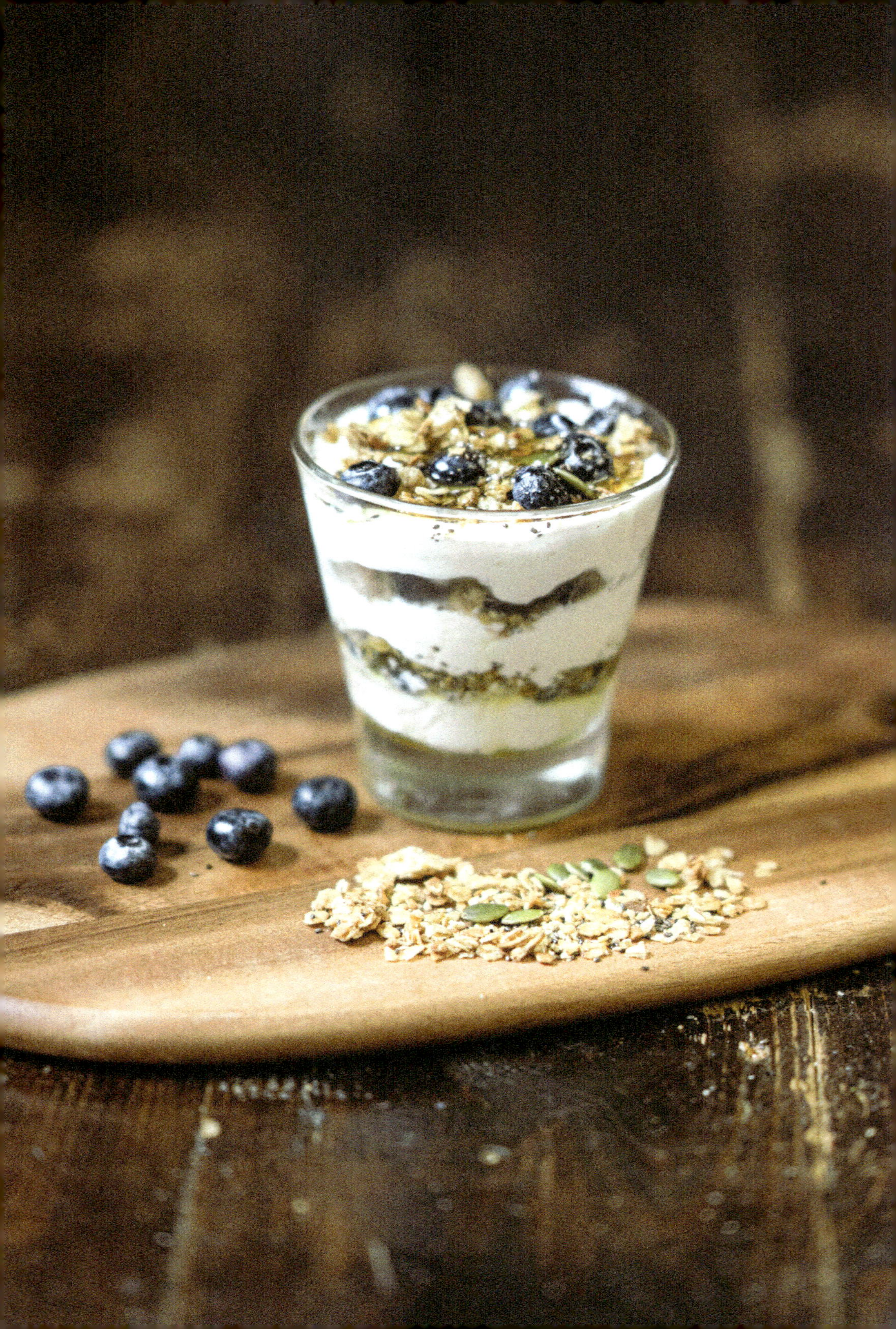

GUT-BOOSTING BERRY YOGHURT PARFAIT

Prep: 15 Mins Chill: 15 mins

Serves 6

1 cup plain, unsweetened Greek yoghurt (rich in probiotics)

1/2 cup mixed berries (blueberries, raspberries, or strawberries)

1 tablespoon ground flaxseeds (high in prebiotic fibre)

2 tablespoons granola (opt for low-sugar varieties)

1 tablespoon chia seeds (another great source of fibre)

1 teaspoon honey or maple syrup (optional for sweetness)

A handful of walnuts (for omega-3s)

This simple, delicious parfait is packed with probiotics from yoghurt and prebiotic fibre from fruit, supporting a healthy gut microbiome.

Instructions

In a small glass or bowl, spoon half of the Greek yoghurt as the base layer.

Add a layer of mixed berries on top of the yoghurt.

Sprinkle half the granola, ground flaxseeds, and chia seeds over the berries.

Repeat the layers with the remaining yoghurt, berries, and granola.

Drizzle honey or maple syrup on top for sweetness, if desired.

Finish with a handful of walnuts for added crunch and omega-3 goodness.

CLEMMIE'S *Tip*

Greek Yoghurt: Provides probiotics to help replenish beneficial bacteria in the gut.

Berries: Rich in antioxidants and fibre, supporting overall gut health.Flaxseeds & Chia Seeds: High in prebiotics, which help feed the good bacteria.

Walnuts: Contain omega-3s, which help reduce inflammation and support gut sunshine for your child's gut garden. They help it grow diverse and strong, which is essential for a healthy immune system. On the other hand, too many processed foods and sugars can disrupt this delicate balance, making it harder for the garden to thrive. This imbalance can leave your child more vulnerable to illness.

Talking to your kids about their gut garden can be fun! Explain that just like a real garden, their gut needs different kinds of 'plants' (bacteria) to stay healthy. Eating a variety of foods helps their garden grow strong, which in turn keeps them healthy and full of energy. This way, they'll understand that when they choose nourishing foods, they're helping their bodies from the inside out!

Antibiotics and other medications are definitely something to keep in mind. While antibiotics can be really important for treating infections, they don't just target the harmful bacteria—they also wipe out some of the good ones too. This can reduce the diversity of your child's gut microbiome, which we know is so vital for their health. Certain antibiotics, like azithromycin, can have an even bigger impact on gut health. That's why it's essential only to use antibiotics when absolutely necessary and prescribed by a doctor.

If your child does need antibiotics, it's worth chatting with a nutritionist about ways to support their gut afterwards. This might include reintroducing beneficial bacteria through food or supplements. Balance is critical here, and nurturing that balance is essential for long-term gut health!

Here's a simple, gut-friendly recipe to help restore beneficial bacteria, especially after antibiotics. It's perfect for breakfast or a snack and supports long-term gut health!

Gut Boosting Berry Yoghurt Parfait

CLEMMIE'S *Tip*

This simple, delicious parfait is packed with probiotics from yoghurt and prebiotic fibre from fruit, supporting a healthy gut microbiome. One of our absolute favourites!

Check our recipes on our YouTube channel or scan the QR code

Here are some fun and engaging ideas for talking to kids about their "gut garden":

CLEMMIE'S *Tip*

Storytime Approach: Create a story about a magical garden where friendly bacteria help plants grow strong. Use characters like "Captain Probiotic" and "Super Fibre" to make it relatable and fun. This can help them understand how good foods support their gut garden.

CLEMMIE'S *Tip*

Garden Metaphors: Explain that just like a garden needs a mix of flowers, vegetables, and sunshine to thrive, their gut needs different foods to stay healthy. Encourage them to think of different foods as "seeds" that help their gut garden grow.

CLEMMIE'S *Tip*

Hands-On Activities: Set up a simple gardening activity where they can plant seeds in pots. Relate this to their gut garden by explaining how they can "plant" good bacteria through healthy foods, just like they are planting seeds in the soil.

CLEMMIE'S *Tip*

Food Colouring Game: Make a game out of choosing colourful fruits and vegetables. Talk about how different colours represent different nutrients and how they help "feed" their gut garden. You could say, "Each colour helps our garden grow bigger and stronger!"

CLEMMIE'S *Tip*

Gut Garden Chart: Create a visual chart together showing their gut garden with pictures of different foods. As they eat various healthy foods, they can add stickers or draw new plants to represent how they're helping their gut garden grow.

CLEMMIE'S *Tip*

Gut Garden Superheroes: Turn foods into superheroes by giving them fun names. For example, "Berry Boosters" for fruits and "Veggie Warriors" for vegetables. This makes it exciting for kids to eat healthy foods, knowing they're like superheroes for their gut.

CLEMMIE'S *Tip*

Cooking Together: Involve them in cooking and preparing meals. Talk about how each ingredient is helping their gut garden grow. For example, say, "These beans are like little helpers for our garden because they're packed with fibre, which feeds the flowers!"

CLEMMIE'S *Tip*

Gut Garden Journal: Encourage them to keep a "Gut Garden Journal" where they can draw or write about the foods they eat each day and how they help their gut garden. This can help them develop an awareness of their food choices.

CLEMMIE'S *Tip*

Songs and Rhymes: Create a fun song or rhyme about the gut garden and the foods that help it thrive. Singing together can make the concept more memorable and enjoyable and don't be embarrassed of you can't sing.

CLEMMIE'S *Tip*

Fun Facts: Share interesting facts about how their gut garden works in simple terms. For example, "Did you know that when you eat yoghurt, you're planting tiny helpers in your gut garden?"

Using these ideas can make the conversation about gut health enjoyable and engaging, helping kids understand the importance of nurturing their "gut garden" in a relatable and fun way!

Beyond diet and medications, stress and lifestyle factors have a significant impact on gut health. Stress can throw the microbiome out of balance, leading to tummy aches or digestive changes. To help your child unwind, consider introducing stress-relieving activities like mindfulness exercises or just getting outside to play.

A consistent sleep routine is also crucial for maintaining a healthy gut. Quality sleep helps support your child's natural body rhythms, including digestion. Plus, regular physical activity can really benefit gut health by keeping the digestive system running smoothly and enhancing overall well-being.

Don't forget about the environment! The world around your child can influence their microbiome in some pretty surprising ways. As a child, I loved making mud potions and spent hours building dens in the garden with my sister; I was constantly covered in mud! Those messy adventures not only filled my days with so much joy but also helped strengthen my immune system. I firmly believe that allowing kids to explore nature, play in the dirt, and interact with the world around them is essential for their health.

Unfortunately, as a nation, we've become too obsessed with baby wipes, bleach, and this idea of 'mess-free play.' Sure, cleanliness is important, but when we focus too much on sanitisation, we're actually limiting our kids' exposure to the beneficial microbes that support their gut health - and missing out on those glorious, muddy memories! Kids need the chance to get grubby, explore, and make a bit of a mess; it's all part of building their resilience and health. So let them splash in that huge puddle and wipe mud on their face.

It's all about finding that sweet spot between hygiene and exposure. Allowing your child to explore different environments can help shape a resilient and adaptable gut microbiome. By keeping these factors in mind, you can support a healthy microbiome for your child, which ultimately contributes to their overall health and happiness!

CLEMMIE'S Tip

One of my absolute favourite books to share with Pia is 'Whiffy Wilson.' It's perfect for teaching kids about the good kind of dirt versus the wrong kind! You can access this books and others I recommend in my Amazon store.

Pre-biotics vs. Pro-biotics

You're at the supermarket, glancing at yoghurt labels, and you spot the words "probiotics" and "prebiotics." You might be wondering what these terms mean and why they're important. Let's break it down.

Probiotics are live bacteria that are great for your gut health. Think of them as friendly soldiers, ready to defend your body against unwanted invaders. They help maintain the balance of microorganisms in your intestines, boosting your immune system and improving digestion. You'll find probiotics in fermented foods such as yoghurt, kefir, sauerkraut, and kimchi.

On the flip side, prebiotics aren't bacteria but are vital for feeding the good bacteria in your gut. They act like fertilisers that help your garden flourish. Prebiotics consist of certain fibres that our bodies can't digest. Instead, they pass through the digestive system, becoming food for the beneficial bacteria. Prebiotics-rich foods include garlic, onions, leeks, asparagus, bananas, and whole grains. Incorporating these into your family's diet can support the growth of healthy bacteria, enhancing overall gut health.

Now, here's where it gets interesting: combining prebiotics and probiotics in your diet can create a powerful synergy. These combinations are known as synbiotic foods, meaning they contain both the good bacteria and the fuel they need to thrive.

Here's a delicious and simple recipe for Banana and Oat Pancakes containing synbiotic foods that you can whip up quickly:

Banana And Oat Pancakes

CLEMMIE'S Tip

This is a simple recipe that features regularly in our morning breakfasts. It is nutritious, very quick to make and impossible to get wrong!

Check our recipes on our YouTube channel or scan the QR code

These pancakes are delicious and a fantastic way to introduce your child to the benefits of prebiotics and probiotics!

If you are looking for an extra protein and fibre boost - I highly recommend Purition wholefood blends; they are not only delicious but are absolutely packed with goodness (also great for hormone balancing, Mums!). You can add them to smoothies, in yoghurt, porridge, cakes and even in cereal - affiliate link.

Pia and I love experimenting in the kitchen together. We often make those banana and oat pancakes, mixing everything up and watching them cook, and I usually let

BANANA AND OAT PANCAKES

Prep: 15 Mins   Cook: 10 Mins (Per batch)

These pancakes are so quic and easy to make. Pia even makes the batter herself now!

Makes 10 pancakes

1 cup rolled oats

1 ripe banana

1/2 cup plain yoghurt (preferably with live cultures)

1/2 cup milk (dairy or non-dairy)

1 teaspoon baking powder

1 teaspoon vanilla extract (optional)

A pinch of salt

Fresh berries (for topping)

Instructions

In a blender or food processor, combine the rolled oats, ripe banana, yoghurt, milk, baking powder, vanilla extract, and salt. Blend until smooth and well combined. The batter should be slightly thick but pourable. If it's too thick, you can add a little more milk to reach your desired consistency.

Heat a non-stick griddle or frying pan over medium heat. You can lightly grease it with a bit of oil or butter if desired.

Pour about 1/4 cup of the pancake batter onto the hot griddle for each pancake. Cook for 2-3 minutes or until bubbles form on the surface and the edges look set. Flip the pancakes and cook for another 1-2 minutes, until golden brown and cooked through.

Remove the pancakes from the griddle and serve them warm, topped with fresh berries for added flavour and nutrition.

Sit down with your little one and enjoy these gut-friendly pancakes together, discussing how the probiotics in the yoghurt and the prebiotic fibres in the oats and banana work together to support your gut health!

CLEMMIE'S Tip

For extra flavour, you can customise the pancakes by adding spices like cinnamon or nutmeg.

Try swapping out the berries for other fruits like sliced bananas or chopped apples or adding a sprinkle of nuts for some crunch

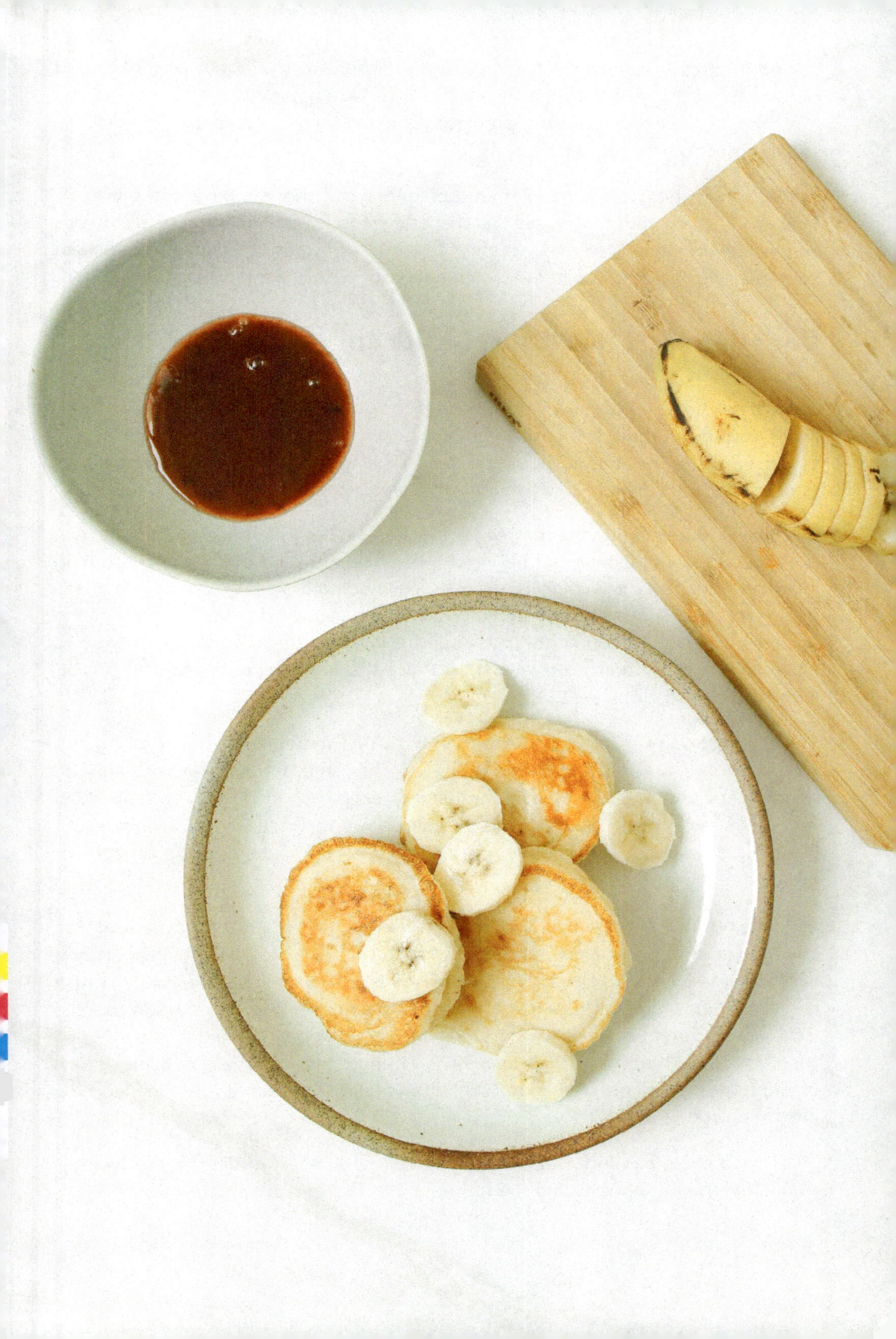

her add her own ingredients (within reason!) When we talk about prebiotics and probiotics, I explain it like this: "Probiotics are like the superheroes in our tummy that help keep us healthy, and prebiotics are the yummy foods that feed those superheroes so they can do their job!"

Remember, the goal is to maintain a balanced diet that supports those friendly bacteria, helping your family feel their best every day. Small, manageable changes can lead to big improvements, whether trying new recipes or adding a banana to your morning cereal; these little adjustments can make a significant difference!

Boosting Gut Health in Children

Lifestyle changes can also work wonders for gut health! Get your kids off their iPads and encourage them to get moving—physical activity is digestion's best friend. Find activities they love, such as a bike ride, a game of tag, or a spontaneous dance show in the living room (we have many of those!).

Never underestimate the power of sleep! A consistent bedtime routine can really do wonders for their gut health. I try to help Pia wind down with a soothing lavender bath and some calming activities like reading or writing together. But let's be honest - this is often easier said than done! Pia usually gets the 'zoomies' in the evening, especially around bath time when she loves to run around the house naked - definitely a girl after my own heart!). If that helps her relax and wear herself out, then who am I to stop her?

I definitely don't want you to think I'm a perfect mother who has it all figured out - I'm right there in the chaos with you! That said, introducing your child to mindfulness practices like deep breathing or simple yoga poses can help them relax and recharge if they struggle to calm down in the evenings. These minor lifestyle adjustments can work wonders alongside their diet, fostering a healthier gut environment.

Here's a fun way to introduce kids to gut health: turn it into an adventure! You can set up a simple science experiment together, like watching how yeast reacts with sugar to create bubbles. It's a playful way to demonstrate fermentation, which is similar to how probiotics function in the gut! You could also create a fun chart to track how different foods affect their mood. Encourage your child to draw happy faces for foods that boost their energy and bring them joy. These activities teach and empower your little ones to make healthy choices for their gut, turning learning into an enjoyable experience!

Let's make gut health fun and engaging for our kids! After all, they're the ones who will carry these habits into the future...but it has to start with us!

Recommended Brands and Products

Diving into the world of probiotics can feel a bit overwhelming with so many options out there. When choosing the right probiotic supplement, there are a few key things to remember. First, go for products that have multiple strains of beneficial bacteria. A diverse range can really amp up the effectiveness! Experts often suggest looking for well-researched strains like Lactobacillus and Bifidobacterium, as they're known for their digestive and immune benefits. Also, check the CFU count (colony-forming units), which tells you how many live bacteria are in each dose. While a higher CFU can be good, remember that more isn't always better—sometimes, a more targeted approach works best. And don't forget to choose products that have been third-party tested. This extra step ensures you get a product that delivers on its promises.

When it comes to kids, age-appropriate probiotics are a must. Young digestive systems are still growing, so selecting probiotics formulated explicitly for them is important. These usually come as chewables, powders, or liquids, which make them easier for kids to take. Plus, they often have lower CFU counts to suit their smaller systems. As you pick a probiotic for your child, keep an eye on any extra ingredients. Many kids' probiotics come flavoured to make them more appealing, but it's wise to avoid those with artificial sweeteners or colours. And definitely check in with a paediatrician before introducing any new supplement to ensure it's a good fit for your child's health.

Stocking your cupboards with prebiotic-rich foods and snacks is another great way to support gut health. Foods such as chicory root, garlic, and onions are fantastic sources, though they aren't exactly what you'd call "snack foods." Think about adding snacks such as whole-grain crackers, apple slices, or a handful of almonds into your child's diet. These snacks not only nourish beneficial gut bacteria but also provide essential nutrients and fibre. When picking packaged snacks, watch out for added sugars or preservatives that can undermine the benefits. Go for minimally processed options that proudly showcase their natural ingredients on the label, which, if I'm completely honest, is extremely hard to find, so you really are better off making them at home (way cheaper, too!).

CLEMMIE'S Tip

Simple Gut-loving Energy Balls

Just 5 ingredients, super easy, and packed with gut-friendly benefits! These are so tempting that we often make a double batch!.

Check our recipes on our YouTube channel or scan the QR code

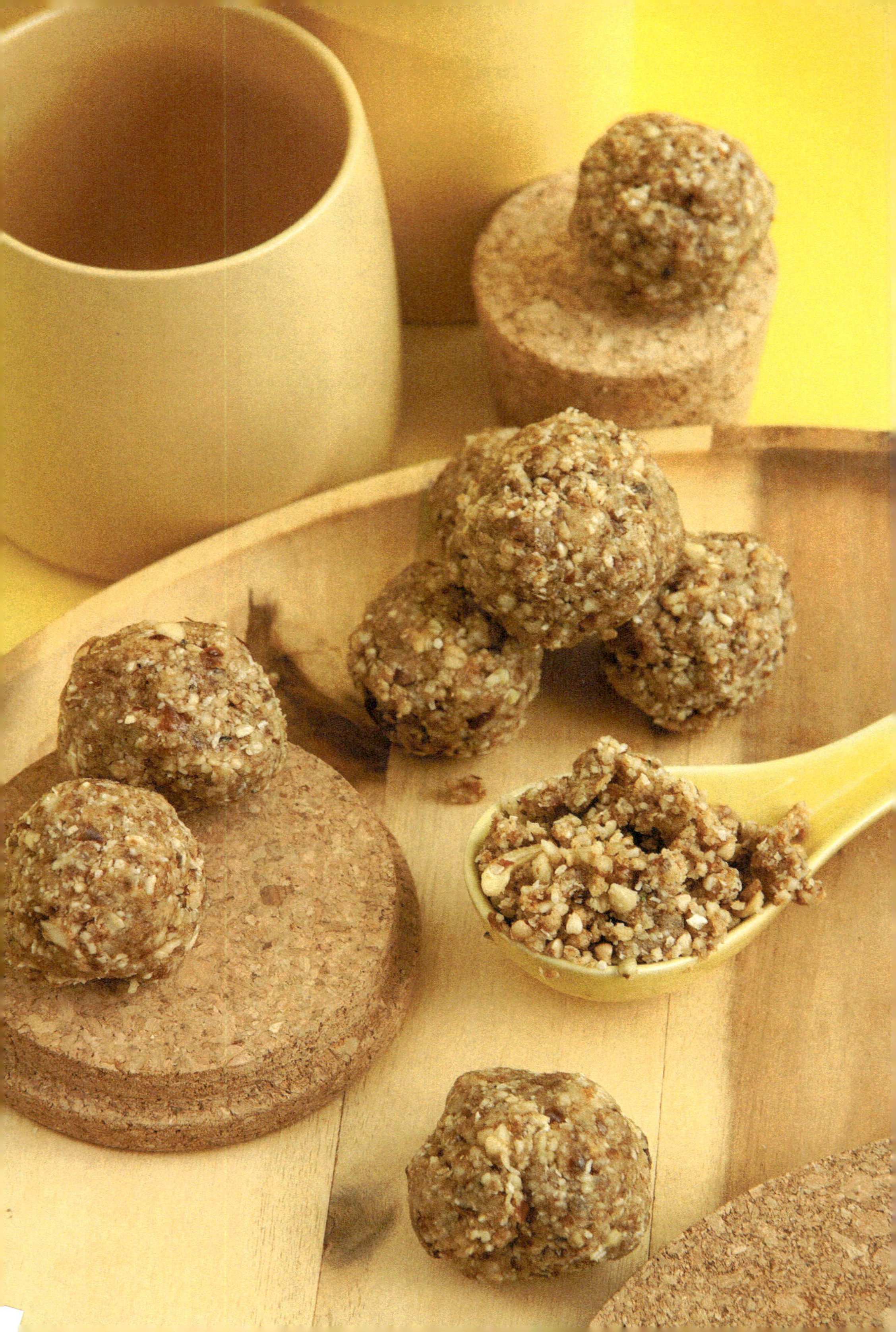

SIMPLE GUT-LOVING ENERGY BALLS

Prep: 15 Mins Chill: 15 mins

These pancakes are so quick and easy to make. Pia even makes the batter herself now!

Makes 20

1 cup oats

½ cup almond butter (or any nut butter)

2 tablespoons honey

½ cup plain Greek yoghurt (for probiotics)

¼ cup ground flaxseeds (for prebiotics)

Instructions

Mix all the ingredients in a bowl until well combined.

Roll the mixture into small balls with your hands.

Refrigerate for 20 minutes to firm up.

Store in the fridge and enjoy!

Being savvy about reading labels can really help you choose gut-friendly products. Look for terms like "live cultures" or "active cultures" in probiotics, which indicate that the product contains those beneficial bacteria. For prebiotics, check that the ingredient list includes chicory root, inulin, or other prebiotic fibres. And be cautious of added sugars and artificial ingredients, as they can cancel out the positive effects you're aiming for. Understanding these labels ensures that the products you choose align with your family's health goals, helping to create a balanced and thriving gut environment.

Oh, and if you're looking to add a protein and fibre boost, I can't recommend Purition wholefood blends enough! They're not just delicious but packed with goodness (perfect for hormone balance, Mums!). You can toss them into smoothies, yoghurt, porridge, cakes, or even sprinkle them on cereal—definitely worth a try! Their contact details and a discount code is in my supplier list in chapter 14.

The Gut-Brain Connection

Imagine your child waking up cheerful and full of energy, ready to take on the day with a smile. For Pia, mornings like that can be hit or miss, especially when we're rushing through the early school run or if she hasn't had a restful night's sleep. But over the years, I've noticed something fascinating—her gut plays a massive role in how her day unfolds. Once I dove deeper into understanding the gut-brain connection, it was like a lightbulb moment. Everything just clicked, and suddenly, it all made sense.

The gut-brain link is like a constant conversation happening inside our bodies. It's not just about digestion; it influences our mood, behaviour, and even how we learn. I've noticed that when Pia's gut is happy and healthy, she's calmer, more focused, and definitely more cooperative with getting ready. But when her guts are out of balance, I can almost tell instantly - she gets irritable or restless, and it's like we're fighting a losing battle before breakfast even begins.

It can be tricky to explain something like the gut-brain connection to a child, but it made a huge difference when I started talking to Pia about it in ways she could relate to. Here are some practical tips that have worked for us

Tips for Talking to Your Kids About the Gut-Brain Connection

CLEMMIE'S Tip

Keep it Simple: Kids don't need the complex science behind the gut-brain axis. I explained it to Pia by saying, "Your tummy talks to your brain. When we feed your tummy good foods, it helps your brain feel happy and strong." Keeping the language basic but fun makes it easier for them to understand.

CLEMMIE'S Tip

Use Fun Analogies: I told Pia to think of her gut like a garden. If we feed it the right 'plants' (good foods), it grows beautifully and makes her feel great. But if we don't take care of it, it gets 'weeds' (bad foods) that can make her tummy and brain feel bad (and a bit sad). You can even let them choose a favourite garden or superhero analogy to make it more engaging!

CLEMMIE'S Tip

Connect it to How They Feel: I'll ask Pia questions like, "Do you remember how you felt super tired and grumpy after eating all that cake at your friend's party?" Then, I'll explain that her tummy wasn't happy because it didn't get the food it needed to feel energised. Relating gut health to her emotions has really helped her connect the dots

CLEMMIE'S Tip

Make it About Empowerment: I always remind Pia that she has the power to make choices that help her gut and brain work together as a team. I'll say, "When you eat foods like yoghurt or oats, it's like giving your brain extra superpowers to help you think better and play longer!" This empowers her to take responsibility and see it as a positive action.

CLEMMIE'S Tip

Make it Visual: Sometimes, I'll show Pia pictures and videos or draw a simple diagram showing how food travels from her tummy to her brain. Seeing this process helps make the connection more tangible, especially for visual learners. You could also create a "gut-brain superhero" together that fights off bad foods and keeps her strong!

CLEMMIE'S Tip

Involve Them in Gut-Healthy Choices: Pia loves being involved in picking out snacks, and now I'll say things like, "Let's choose a snack that's going to help your brain feel great today." We'll talk about which foods support her tummy, like yoghurt for probiotics or bananas for fibre. This way, she feels part of the process and understands the benefits.

Disclaimer: I still let Pia have chocolate and cake because, let's be honest, who doesn't love cake? I want her to enjoy life and all the sweet moments that come with it. For me, it's not about restriction—it's about planting little seeds of nutrition education along the way so that when she's older, she'll naturally make healthier choices while still indulging in the treats she loves. Because it's all about balance, right?

By talking about the gut-brain connection in ways that are relatable to Pia, it's become much easier to help her understand why certain foods are good for her and why routines like bedtime are so important. Plus, it's turned into a fun, engaging way to chat about nutrition and health without feeling like I'm nagging or lecturing!

Helping your child understand the gut-brain connection is all about setting them up for a healthier, happier life. They can make mindful choices and actually feel the benefits—whether it's better focus at school or just starting the day in a great mood. My book is about giving our kids the knowledge to fuel themselves so that when they're old enough to cook for themselves, they actually understand how nutrition works. Honestly, what a gift that is!

What to do Next

1. Stock up for our gut-friendly recipes - check your cupboards for ingredients for our Berry Yoghurt Parfait and Energy Balls. These are absolute lifesavers for busy days!
2. Start your "Gut Garden Chart" - grab some fun stickers and let the kids track their gut-friendly foods. Pia loves putting a star next to each new food she tries!
3. Make probiotics part of your daily routine - whether it's yoghurt at breakfast or trying some kid-friendly kefir. Take baby steps and make it fun!
4. Add prebiotic foods to your weekly shop - things like bananas, onions, and whole grains. These feed our good gut bacteria (or as we call them, our "tummy superheroes").
5. Get outside and get dirty - plan some outdoor adventures. Play with the pets and have some old fashioned fun. Remember, a little dirt is good for building strong gut health!
6. Create a gut-friendly bedtime routine - consistent timing and calming activities make such a difference to both sleep and digestion.
7. Try some simple "gut science" experiments with the kids - making these concepts fun and visual helps them understand why gut health matters.
8. Make a visual gut-brain connection chart with your little ones - we love

Chapter Six

Meal Prep and Planning for Busy Families

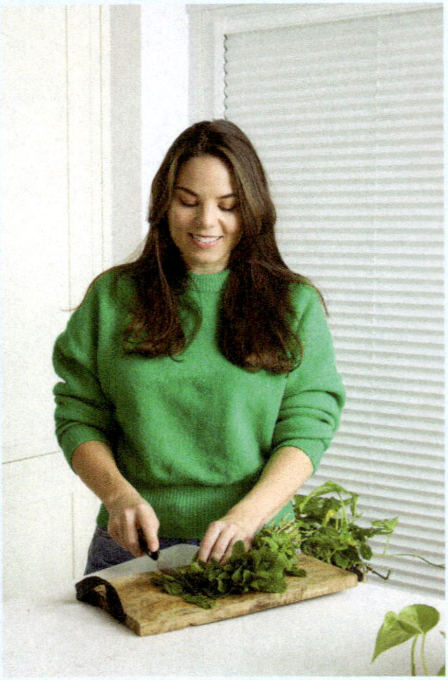
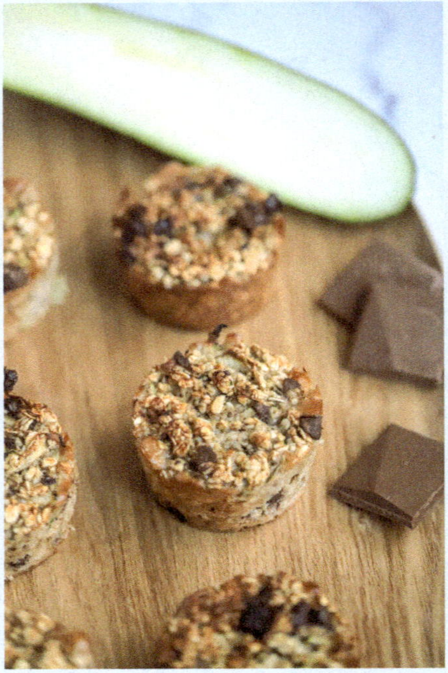
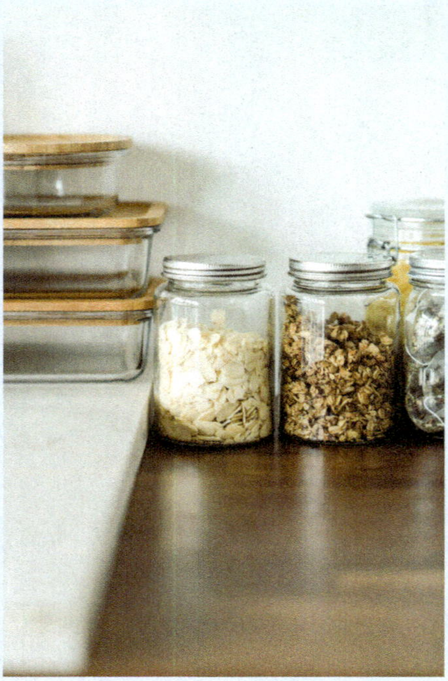
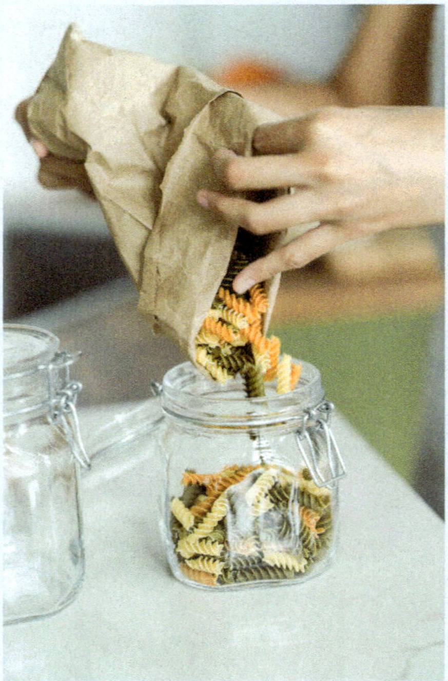

Meal Prep and Planning for Busy Families

It's a typical Monday morning, and I'm doing my best impression of an octopus whilst making pancakes, packing lunches, hunting for missing shoes, and trying to remember if it's PE day and if I actually turned on the washing machine. Sound familiar? This chaotic routine is exactly why meal prepping has been a lifesaver for my sanity (and likely why I haven't resorted to ordering takeaway five nights a week!).

The Meal Prep Revolution

I used to think meal prepping was something only super-organised people did - those Instagram-perfect mums with their colour-coded containers and perfectly aligned spice racks. Meanwhile, I was scrambling at 6 p.m., staring into the fridge as if it might magically produce dinner if I looked hard enough.

Meal prepping isn't about being perfect; it's about being practical. I realised this one chaotic weekday evening when I got home late from work. Pia was hungry, tired, and on the verge of a meltdown - a delightful combination. I went to grab the chicken I thought I'd left to defrost, only to find it still rock-hard in the freezer. With no backup options, no patience, and a hungry child on my hands, I gave in and ordered pizza. That night, exhausted and a little defeated, I knew something had to change.

Every Sunday afternoon or sometimes Monday, if the weekend doesn't go as planned, I set aside a few hours to prepare simple dinners for the week (and breakfasts if I'm feeling exceptionally organised). It saves me time in the evenings, ensures we eat a variety of balanced meals throughout the week and makes me feel like a supermum!

The Great Container Adventure

Let's briefly discuss meal-prep tools because they can make or break your prep game. I learned this the hard way after a ginormous soup explosion last year—not all containers are created equal, especially when it comes to hot soup in a bag!

First things first: good containers are worth their weight in gold. I discovered this after finding mysterious purple stains in my handbag from a leaking beetroot container during a work meeting. I'm now officially obsessed with BPA-free containers or, ideally, glass containers that actually seal properly (I have listed those suppliers I really rate in chapter 14). Pia calls them our "treasure boxes" because they keep our food safe like little treasure chests—whatever works!

A slow cooker or Instant Pot are absolute game-changers. I was sceptical at first - another kitchen gadget to take up space and gather dust. But now I want to write love songs about my slow cooker. Last week, I threw in some chicken, vegetables, and stock before the school run, and by dinner time, we had this fantastic stew that made me look like a domestic goddess. Pia even asked if I'd been cooking all day!

Let's talk about knives for a minute. No one has time to spend 20 minutes trying to cut a butternut squash with a butter knife. Life's too short for blunt knives. I invested in a good chef's knife and a proper cutting board, and suddenly, meal prep wasn't a workout anymore.

The Sunday Prep Party

Our Sunday prep sessions have become a whole thing now. We blast music (currently rotating between Disney songs and my Ibiza chillout playlist) and turn the kitchen into a "food factory." Here's how it typically goes:

2 PM: Start with what Pia calls "vegetable surgery" - chopping all our veggies for the week

3 PM: Move on to batch cooking grains (usually while having a dance break)

4 PM: Prep proteins and put together any make-ahead meals

5 PM: Package everything up (this is where those treasure box containers come in!)

However, I should mention that this timeline is more of a rough guide. Last Sunday, we spent an extra 20 minutes pretending our wooden spoons were microphones while singing "Let It Go".

Breakfast Heroes

Trying to make a proper breakfast while finishing homework, finding PE kits, and remembering to feed the cat (sorry, Rupert!) is an Olympic sport. That's why these make-ahead breakfasts have become my secret weapons.

Overnight Oats Recipe

CLEMMIE'S Tip

Overnight oats are a lifesaver when you're juggling a million things in the morning! Plus, you can prep them in minutes the night before—no cooking required—just mix and go.

Check our recipes on our YouTube channel or scan the QR code

Quick n Easy Pancake Recipe

CLEMMIE'S Tip

Our weekend mornings wouldn't be complete without these easy pancakes! They're light, fluffy, and sneakily healthy. You can even make a big batch and freeze them for a quick weekday breakfast—just pop them in the toaster to reheat!

Check our recipes on our YouTube channel or scan the QR code

Breakfast Burritos

CLEMMIE'S Tip

These are my go-to for mad rush mornings when everyone's running out the door! You can make these ahead and wrap them in foil—great for busy mornings when you're racing out the door in a panic!

Check our recipes on our YouTube channel or scan the QR code

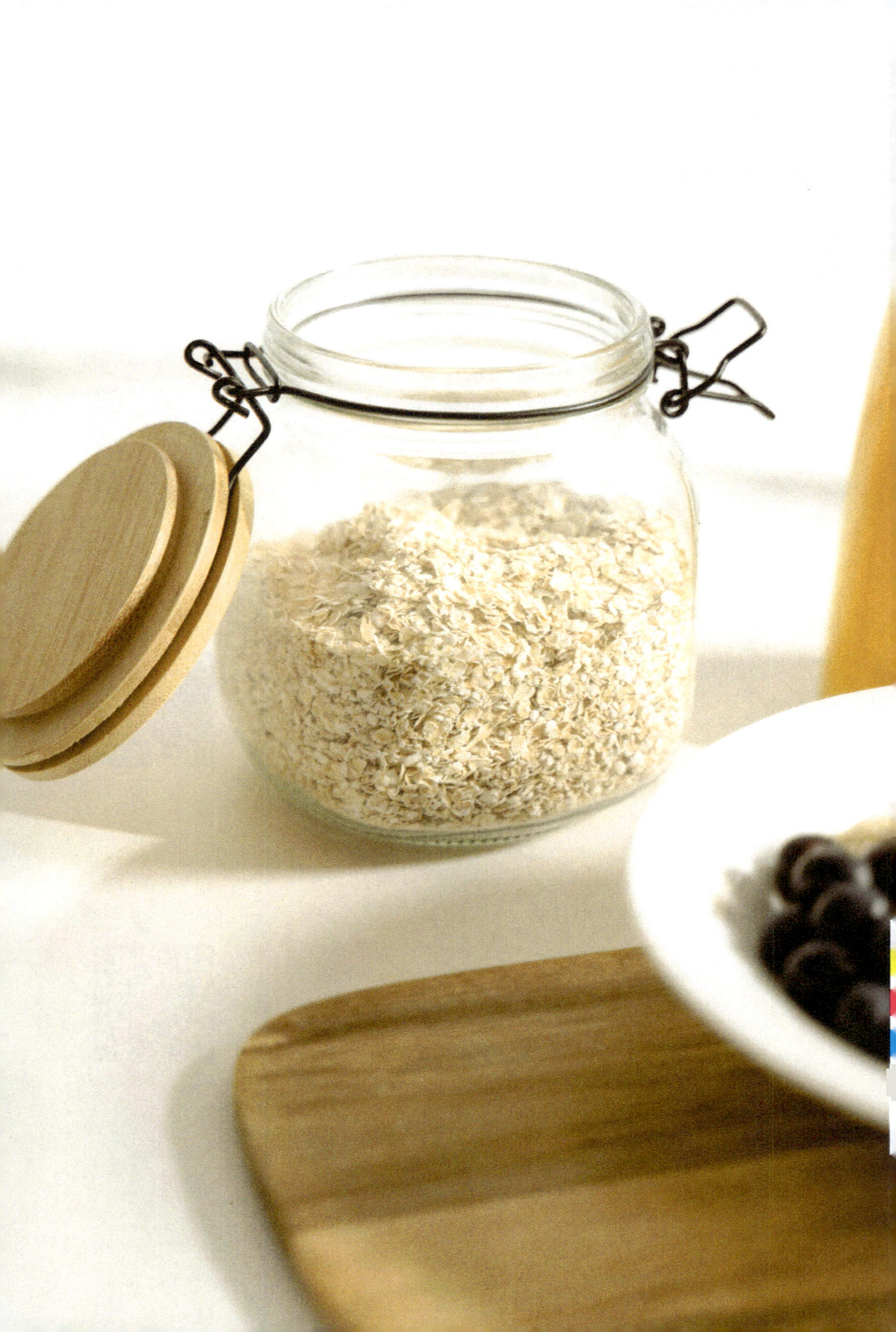

OVERNIGHT OATS

Serves 1

Prep: 5 Mins   Chill: 6 hours

½ cup oats

½ cup milk (or any dairy-free option, like almond or oat milk)

2 tbsp chia seeds

1 tsp honey or maple syrup

¼ tsp vanilla extract (optional)

Topping Ideas:

Fresh berries or chopped banana (Pia loves to help pick the toppings!)

A dollop of yoghurt

A sprinkle of nuts, seeds, or a handful of granola for crunch

Overnight oats are a lifesaver when you're juggling a million things in the morning! Plus, you can prep them in minutes the night before—no cooking required—just mix and go.

Instructions

Add the dates, oats, walnuts, flax, vanilla cinnamon Simply stir the base ingredients together in a jar or bowl, cover, and leave in the fridge overnight.

In the morning, add your toppings.

The best part? You can mix it up however you like. Sometimes, I sneak in some grated courgette or a spoonful of nut butter for extra goodness!

QUICK 'N EASY PANCAKES

Makes 8–10
Serves 2–3

Prep: 5 Mins Cook: 10 Mins (Per batch)

1 cup self-raising flour (or whole wheat for a fibre boost)

1 egg

1 cup milk (or a dairy-free option)

1 mashed banana (sweetens naturally)

A pinch of cinnamon (blood sugar balancing)

Our weekend mornings wouldn't be complete without these easy pancakes that even Pia loves! They're light, fluffy, and sneakily healthy.

Instructions

Whisk all the ingredients together until smooth.

Heat a little butter or oil in a pan over medium heat.

Drop spoonfuls of the batter into the pan and cook until bubbles appear on the surface. Flip and cook for another 1-2 minutes.

Serve with fresh fruit or a drizzle of honey.

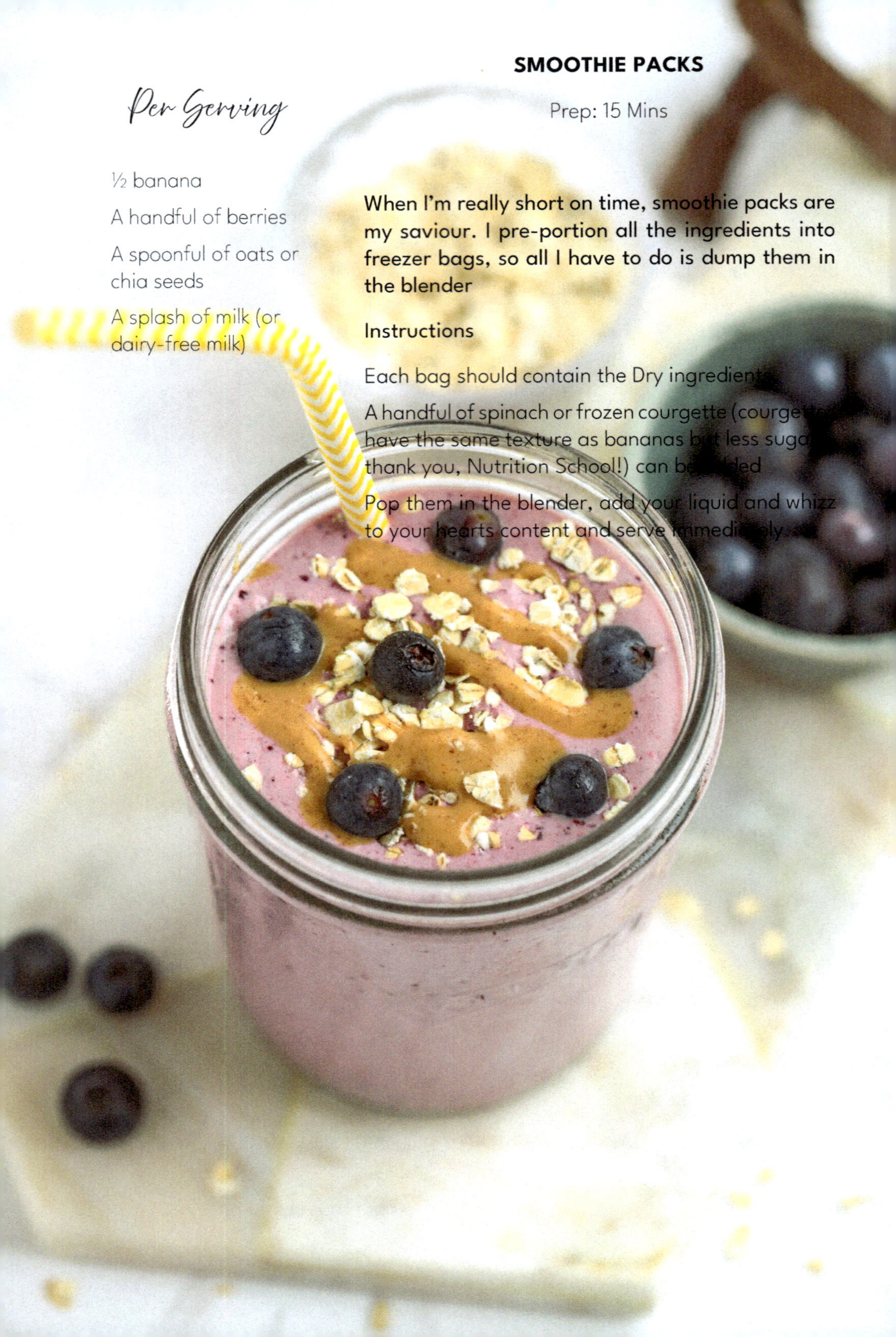

SMOOTHIE PACKS

Prep: 15 Mins

Per Serving

½ banana

A handful of berries

A spoonful of oats or chia seeds

A splash of milk (or dairy-free milk)

When I'm really short on time, smoothie packs are my saviour. I pre-portion all the ingredients into freezer bags, so all I have to do is dump them in the blender

Instructions

Each bag should contain the Dry ingredients

A handful of spinach or frozen courgette (courgettes have the same texture as bananas but less sugar – thank you, Nutrition School!) can be added

Pop them in the blender, add your liquid and whizz to your hearts content and serve immediately

7 MINUTE BREAKFAST BURRITOS

Prep: 2 Mins   Cook: 5 Mins

Per Serving

2 eggs

A handful of grated cheese

1 wrap

Optional: spinach, avocado slices, or leftover veggies

These are my go-to for mad rush mornings when everyone's running out the door! They're quick, easy, and packed with protein to keep us all going until lunch.

Instructions

Scramble the eggs in a non-stick pan.

Add cheese and any extras like spinach or avocado.

Wrap it all up in the tortilla, and you're done!

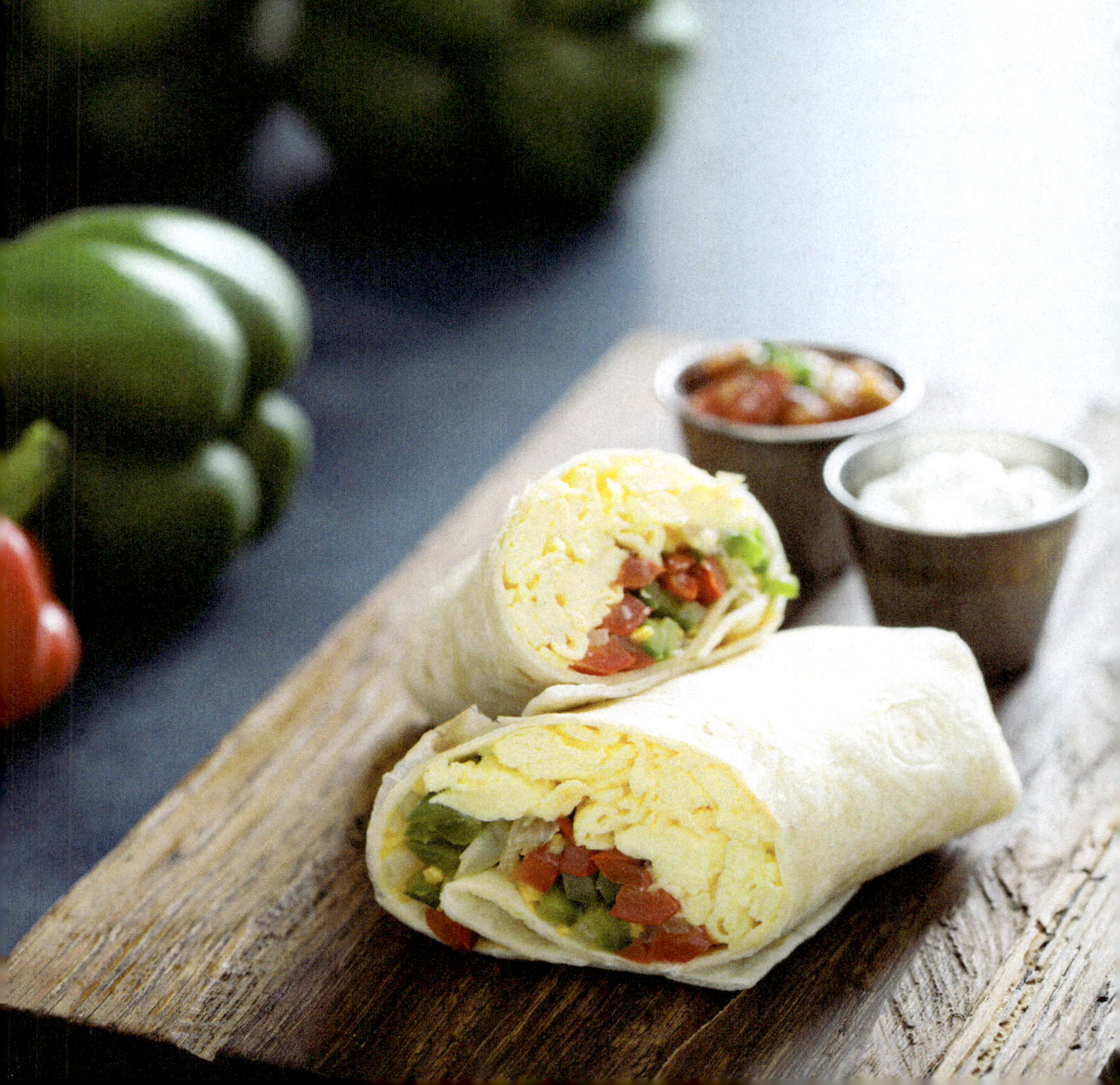

Smoothie Packs

CLEMMIE'S *Tip*

When I'm really short on time, smoothie packs are my saviour. I pre-portion all the ingredients into freezer bags, so all I have to do is dump them in the blender.

Check our recipes on our YouTube channel or scan the QR code

Pia loves to pick the fruits—and I always sneak in a veggie or two! Blend everything together, and you have a nutritious breakfast or snack in seconds! These are perfect for when we need something quick but still healthy. I've a whole separate book on great smoothie recipes that you can download from Amazon.

Pia loves creating her own little breakfast menu, and I've found it takes some pressure off me and teaches her a little independence, too. I sometimes set up a little "breakfast station" in the kitchen where she can reach everything herself. It's like her own personal breakfast café, and she's in charge of making it happen. Watching her pick out her favourite fruit or grab some yoghurt makes me feel like maybe, just maybe, I'm nailing this parenting thing.

At the end of the day (or the beginning, I guess), breakfast is more than just food. It's those little moments of connection before we all head out in different directions. Whether it's laughing over a bowl of porridge or squeezing in a quick chat while blending a smoothie, those small moments mean everything. Life gets busy, but taking time to nourish both body and soul with something as simple as breakfast? That's where the magic is.

Lunchbox Magic

You know you're a parent when you buy heart-shaped sandwich cutters at midnight on Amazon. But honestly, the day I discovered that Pia would eat an entire sandwich if it was cut into a teddy bear shape was like winning the lottery.

Speaking of lunch prep, let's talk about expectations versus reality for a minute. Those Instagram-worthy bento boxes with food art that look like actual masterpieces? Yeah, I tried that exactly once. I spent an hour making a panda face out of rice and seaweed, only for Pia to come home and tell me it looked more like a sad bear who needed a nap and that green stuff stunk. Now, I go for a more "achievable cute" - think star-shaped cucumbers and heart-shaped sandwiches. Manageable but still special enough to make her smile when she opens her lunchbox.

The Dinner Dash

That dreaded moment when you realise it's dinner time, and you haven't even thought about what to cook. Familiar? I used to have a minor panic attack every day at 5:30 PM until I got organised and created a list of simple meals I could throw together in 30 minutes or less, using stuff I always have in the fridge or freezer.

Here's a real story from last week: I'd completely lost track of time during a work call, and suddenly, it was 5:45 p.m. Pia was doing her homework at the kitchen table, getting hangrier by the minute.. But because I had prepped some basics on Sunday, I managed to throw together a rice bowl that she actually ate. Pre-cooked rice, some chopped veggies, leftover chicken, and "magic sauce" (just yoghurt with a bit of honey and lemon).

The Reality Check

Look, I need to be honest here. Even with all this prep and planning, sometimes things go sideways. Last month, I had a week's worth of beautifully prepped and organised meals. I felt like I had it all together. Then, our fridge decided to have a midlife crisis and stopped working. Cue emergency fish finger dinner and a very smug cat who got to eat a lot of defrosting chicken!

But you know what? That's real life. Sometimes your beautiful meal prep plans fall apart, sometimes the kids decide they no longer eat anything green, and sometimes you just don't have the energy to be super organised. And that's completely okay!

The whole point of meal prepping isn't to add more pressure to our already busy lives—it's to make things easier. Even if all you manage to do in one week is chop some vegetables and cook a batch of rice, that's still a win. As I always say to Pia, "Perfect is boring; progress is exciting!"

Making It All Work

While I'm doing the main prep, I deliberately make extra of everything. I double up on roasted vegetables and hide them in pasta sauces. The chicken I'm cooking for sandwiches gets shredded and frozen for emergency quesadillas. It means that I can produce dinner in 10 minutes flat.

Pia is slowly starting to help me more during our prep sessions, though "helping" might be a stretch. Last Sunday, she was busy "helping" me pack vegetables into containers, and I noticed she'd arranged them all into smiley faces. It wasn't exactly efficient, but it kept her entertained for a solid hour. I have found that she's actually more likely to eat the vegetables she's helped prepare, even if they end up a little squashed from being rearranged seventeen times.

The Storage Solution

Organising my fridge has been a game-changer. I used to just shove all my prepped food in wherever it would fit, only to spend ages hunting for things later. Now, thanks to some handy fridge organisers from Amazon, everything has its place. I've divided the fridge into zones: ready-to-eat snacks at kid height, prepped ingredients on the middle shelf, and backup supplies at the back.

For those who want to take it a step further, labelling items with day-of-the-week stickers sounds ideal in theory. But if you miss a day, it can quickly get confusing and create more admin.

The Emergency Backup Plan

Nobody talks about your meal prep backup plan enough. For those weeks when everything goes wrong and you can't finish your usual prep, I keep portions of cooked rice, frozen vegetables, and some emergency protein options. It's saved dinner more times than I can count.

Last month, when I had a terrible cold and couldn't face my usual Sunday prep session, this kit was an absolute lifesaver. Although the meals weren't as varied and exciting as our usual ones, everyone was fed nutritious food without me having to think too hard.

Sometimes, the washing still gets left in the machine, the pancakes still get burnt, and dinner might occasionally be eggs on toast. We're all just doing our best. And if meal prepping helps make our weeks a little easier and our meals a little healthier, then I count that as a win - even if my vegetable-chopping skills will never make it onto MasterChef!

What to Do Next

1. Start small—don't try to prep a whole week's worth of meals right away. Begin by chopping vegetables for two days and work up from there.
2. Create your own backup meal plan by stocking your freezer with two to three emergency meals. You can always gook extra in your prep sessions and just put them in the freezer.
3. Invest in good containers. Check my Amazon shop for the ones that have survived Pia's "accidental drop tests" (and my questionable stacking abilities)..

4. Double up recipes and store extras for the days when you just don't have the time (or energy) to cook from scratch. Look for deals at the supermarket where they have 2-for-1 offers

5. Set up your child-friendly prep station. Get those safe knives and create a space where kids can help without chaos. There are some great options outlines in my supplier list n chapter 14.

6. Organise your fridge with zones. My 'Meal prep + fridge organisation' list is available on my Amazon shop but you can always just make your own.

7. Batch-cook your breakfast basics. Start with our overnight oats or pancake recipes and build from there.

Chapter 7

Making Nutrition Fun and Educational

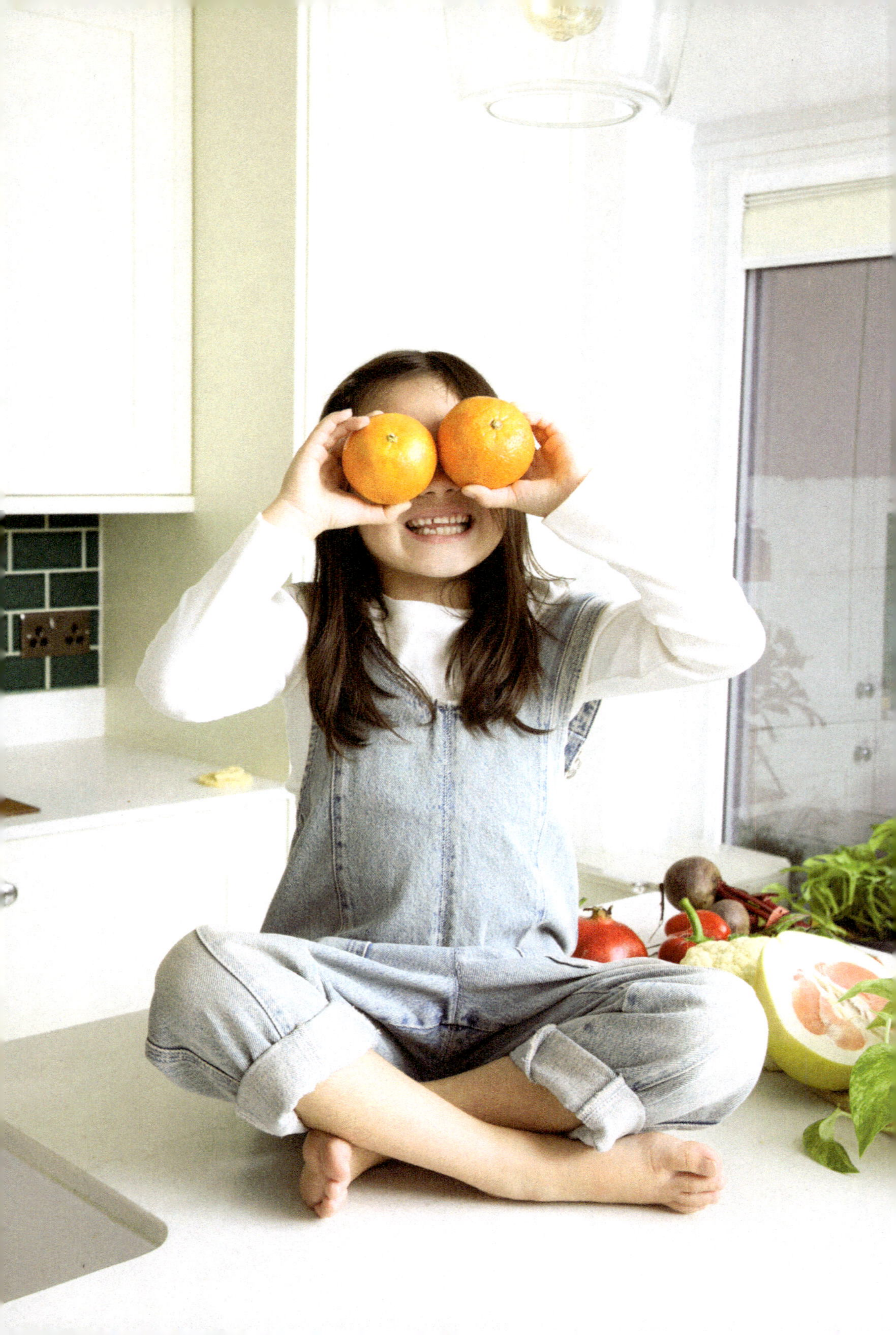

Making Nutrition Fun and Educational

You know those rainy days when the kids are bouncing off the walls, and you're desperately trying not to resort to screen time? Last Wednesday was one of those days. Pia was doing her best impression of a hurricane in the living room, and I could feel that familiar panic rising - the "how am I going to entertain her for the next four hours?" panic that every parent knows too well. That's when I remembered something my mother used to do with me: she'd turn ordinary moments into stories.

The Birth of Our Food Heroes

We were having one of those epic mealtime battles about broccoli (you know, the ones). In complete desperation, I started telling Pia about "Benny the Bold Broccoli", a brave little vegetable with superpowers. I'll be honest; I was making it up as I went along and half expecting eye rolls. But something magical happened. She not only ate the broccoli but asked to hear more about Benny's adventures.

That's when "Sammy the Strong Strawberry" joined our little food superhero universe. Sammy wasn't just any strawberry - oh no, he was a brave little fruit with a passion for healthy eating and a special power to make anyone who ate him super strong. Before I knew it, Pia was creating her own characters. "Carla, the Cute Carrot" was her invention, complete with night-vision powers "because carrots help you see in the dark, right, Mummy?"

Our latest food hero adventure was meant to be a simple story about trying new foods, but it turned into this elaborate tale involving Sammy the Strawberry travelling around the world. Pia was so invested that she insisted on creating passports for all our fruit and vegetable heroes. We spent the entire afternoon drawing stamps from different countries and talking about what foods our heroes might try in each place. Who knew a rainy day could turn into such a delicious geography lesson?

When Food Stories Go Wrong

I should probably tell you about some of our less successful attempts, too, because of course not everything works out as planned! For example, I once tried to introduce "Peter the Powerful Pea" and accidentally knocked the entire bowl of peas onto the floor. Pia found it hilarious and now insists that Peter's superpower is "escape and roll"!

Or the time our attempt at a "Cooking with Mummy" session ended with what I can only describe as a flour explosion. The kitchen looked like a snowstorm had hit it, and our vegetable smoothie tasted suspiciously like grass. But do you know what? Pia still talks about that day as one of her favourites. Sometimes, the messiest moments make the best memories!

Around the World in 80 Bites

We once turned our kitchen into an "International Food Airport" and made passports for our food heroes, complete with little stamps and visas (basically stickers). Our first stop was Japan, where Sammy the Strawberry tried sushi for the first time. Of course, this meant WE had to try making sushi too. Picture me trying to roll a bamboo mat while Pia enthusiastically scattered rice everywhere, declaring that she was "making it snow in Japan".

The best part about these food adventures is how they spark the most amazing conversations. While we were making our slightly wonky sushi rolls, Pia asked why Japanese children eat different breakfasts from us. This led to this wonderful discussion about different food cultures and how what seems strange to us might be completely normal to someone else. Though I'm not entirely sure she was convinced about the idea of having soup for breakfast!

Technology: Friend or Foe?

Let's talk about screen time for a minute because I know we all struggle with it. Yes, I'm a nutritionist, and yes, I sometimes let Pia play on the iPad while I'm cooking dinner. But I've learned to be strategic about it. We've found some fantastic apps that actually make learning about nutrition fun (and give me those precious 20 minutes to get dinner started).

The other day, Pia was playing with this food education app called 'This is my food' when she suddenly called, "Mummy, did you know that carrots have beta-carotene? That's what makes them orange!" I nearly dropped the spatula—partly because I was surprised to hear my 7-year-old say 'beta-carotene' and partly because I realised these apps were actually teaching her something useful!

Themed Food Days

Our themed food days started as a way to make weekday dinners more exciting, but they've turned into elaborate productions that Pia now plans days in advance. Italian Night has always been my favourite, although flipping pizza dough is harder than it looks on YouTube. We ended up with dough stuck to the ceiling for weeks!

We did, however, make a delicious (and healthy!) vanilla gelato that's now become a staple on Italian Night:

CLEMMIE'S Tip

Vanilla Banana Nice-Cream

This vanilla nice cream is a healthy, creamy treat that's perfect for satisfying your sweet tooth. The addition of vanilla protein powder not only thickens the nice cream but also boosts its protein content, making it an even more nutritious option. Feel free to experiment with different add-ins like cocoa powder or nut butter for a twist!

Check our recipes on our YouTube channel or scan the QR code

This vanilla nice cream is a healthy, creamy treat that's perfect for satisfying your sweet tooth. The addition of vanilla protein powder not only thickens the nice cream but also boosts its protein content, making it an even more nutritious option. Feel free to experiment with different add-ins like cocoa powder or nut butter for a twist.

The real magic of these themed nights isn't just in the food, though - it's in the conversations they spark. During our Mexican Fiesta Night, while Pia was enthusiastically mashing avocados, we talked about how ancient Aztecs used to grow their food on floating gardens. Her mind was blown! Now she's convinced we should turn our porch into a "floating garden" - I'm still trying to figure out how to explain the logistics of that one!

Visual Learning

Our fridge has become this ever-changing exhibition of food art. We started with a simple rainbow chart showing different fruits and vegetables, but it's evolved into

VANILLA BANANA NICE CREAM

Prep: 5 Mins Freezing 2 hours (for Bananas)

Total Time: Approximately 2 hours 5 minutes

This vanilla nice cream is a healthy, creamy treat that's perfect for satisfying your sweet tooth. The addition of vanilla protein powder not only thickens the nice cream but also boosts its protein content, making it an even more nutritious option. Feel free to experiment with different add-ins like cocoa powder or nut butter for a twist!

Serves 2

2 ripe bananas, sliced and frozen

1 teaspoon vanilla extract

1-2 tablespoons milk (dairy or non-dairy, as desired)

1 scoop vanilla protein powder (optional for added thickness and protein)

Optional toppings: chopped nuts, chocolate chips, fresh fruit, or coconut flakes

Instructions

Prepare the Bananas: If you haven't already, slice the ripe bananas and freeze them for at least 2 hours or until completely frozen.

Blend the Ingredients: In a food processor or blender, combine the frozen banana slices, vanilla extract, and vanilla protein powder (if using).

Add Milk: Blend until smooth, scraping down the sides as needed. If the mixture is too thick, add 1 tablespoon of milk at a time until you reach your desired consistency.

Serve: Once smooth and creamy, serve immediately for a soft-serve texture, or transfer to an airtight container and freeze for about 30 minutes for a firmer nice cream.

Add Toppings: Top with your favourite toppings, like nuts, chocolate chips, or fresh fruit.

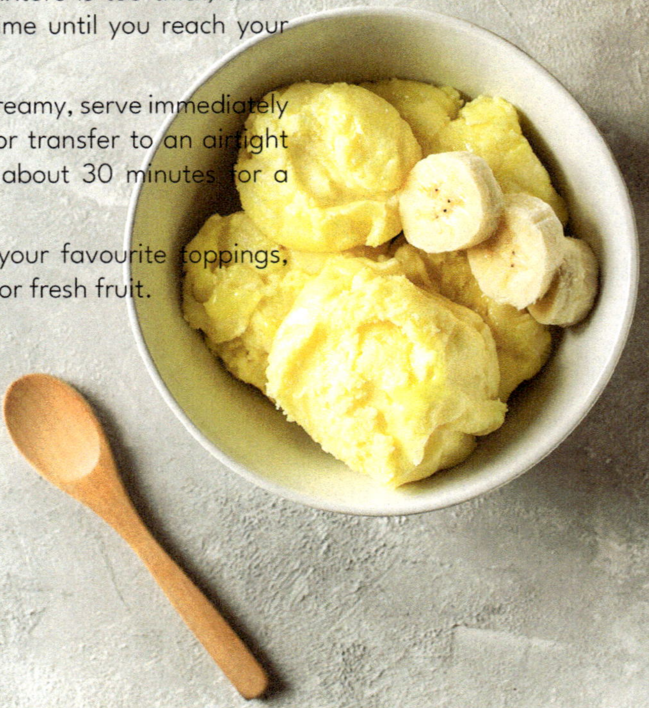

this massive collage of Pia's food hero artwork, pictures of meals we've tried, and our "adventure maps" showing where different foods come from.

The other day, Pia created a "Superhero Food Journal"—an adorable mix of drawings and stickers where she tracks her daily "power foods." According to her latest entry, strawberries give her "super speed," and spinach makes her "strong like a tiger." I haven't had the heart to correct her on that last one—honestly, whatever gets her eating more greens.

Body Image and Food Stories

The other day, something happened that really stopped me in my tracks. Pia came home from school and asked if certain foods would make her "fat". She's seven—SEVEN! Hearing that word hurt my heart, and it reminded me exactly why the way we talk about food is so incredibly important.

Instead of panicking (okay, I panicked a little), I brought out our food heroes. We chatted about how Sammy the Strawberry never talks about foods making you fat or thin - instead, he talks about how different foods give you different powers. Carrots help you see in the dark; beans provide you with energy for playing, and berries help your brain solve puzzles. Watching her face light up as we discussed all these "superpowers" reminded me that children naturally want to learn how food helps them, not how it might harm them.

This is something I feel really passionate about, both as a nutritionist and as a mum. When we focus our food conversations on strength, energy and fun rather than size or restrictions, we help build a foundation for a healthy relationship with food that can last a lifetime. Though I must admit, Pia now insists on eating bananas before her dance class because "they give me super jumping powers" - not quite scientifically accurate, but I'll take it!

Numbers Matter

Did you know that only 18% of children aged 5-15 in the UK are eating their five-a-day? As a nutritionist, that statistic worries me. As a mum, it breaks my heart. But here's the thing - throwing these numbers at kids or trying to force-feed them vegetables isn't the answer. Trust me, I've tried (and failed) that approach!

Instead, I've found that making food fun and educational really does work. When Pia learned that Roman gladiators ate mainly vegetables (yes, I might have embellished this historical fact slightly), suddenly, her vegetables became "gladiator food". Sometimes, it's these silly little reframes that make all the difference.

The Kitchen Laboratory

One rainy afternoon last week, our kitchen turned into a "Food Science Lab". We were learning about why apples go brown when you cut them (thanks to a school science project), and somehow, this turned into a full-blown experiment testing different fruits and vegetables. Did you know that if you squeeze lemon juice on apple slices, they don't turn brown? Pia thought this was actual magic and now refers to lemons as "the wizard fruit".

These moments of discovery are precious, not just because they teach her about food but also because they create memories. Yes, sometimes our experiments go wrong, but even the disasters become part of our story.

What To Do Next

1. Start your own Food Hero stories - don't worry about being perfect! Get your child to come up with some silly names. I guarantee there will be fits of giggles.

2. Create a Food Hero passport for your kitchen adventures. Let your little ones decorate it and add "stamps" for each new food they try.

3. Plan your first themed food night - keep it simple! Maybe start with Italian (our Vanilla Nice Cream recipe is perfect for this) or Mexican (guacamole is always a winner, even if it ends up everywhere).

4. Download our recommended apps for rainy days - I've put together a list of the ones that actually work (and won't drive you crazy with annoying sound effects).

5. Start a simple food journal with your child - make it fun with stickers and drawings. Focus on "superpowers" rather than good or bad foods.

6. Create your own kitchen science experiment. My blog has simple, safe ideas that teach kids about nutrition while having fun but a quick search will also yield masses of videos.

7. Make a rainbow chart for your fridge. Get the kids involved in the artwork, and use it to track your colourful food adventures.

8. Join the dedicated Facebook group, for readers of this book where parents share their food hero stories and creative ideas. Sometimes, the best inspiration comes from other parents in the trenches!

Chapter Eight

Overcoming Resistance from Family Members

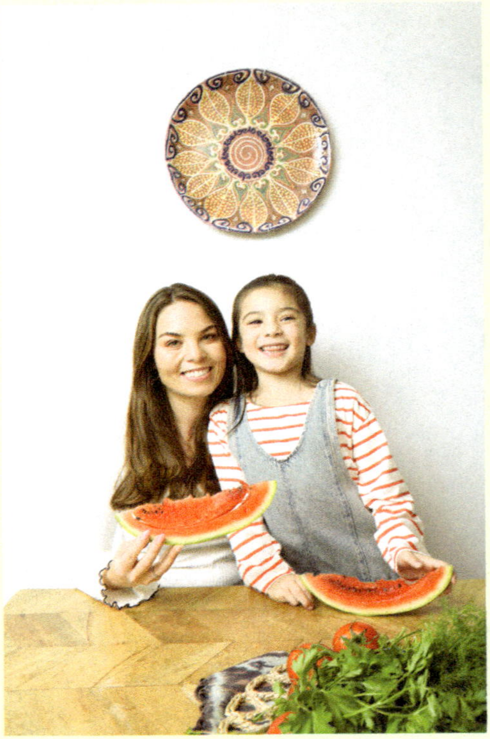
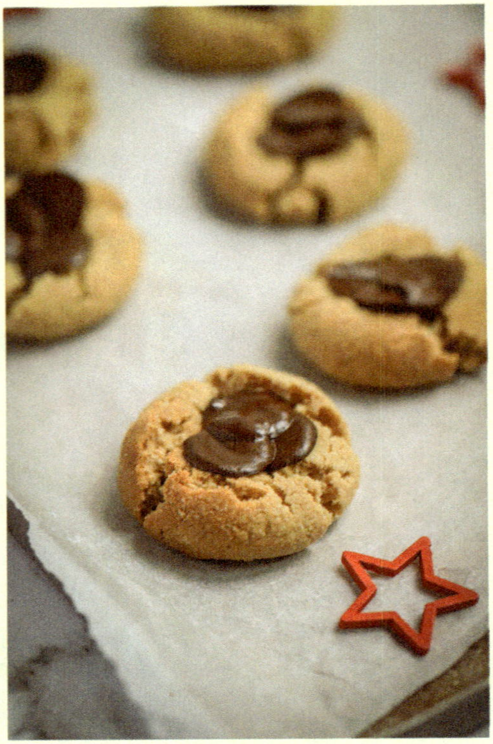
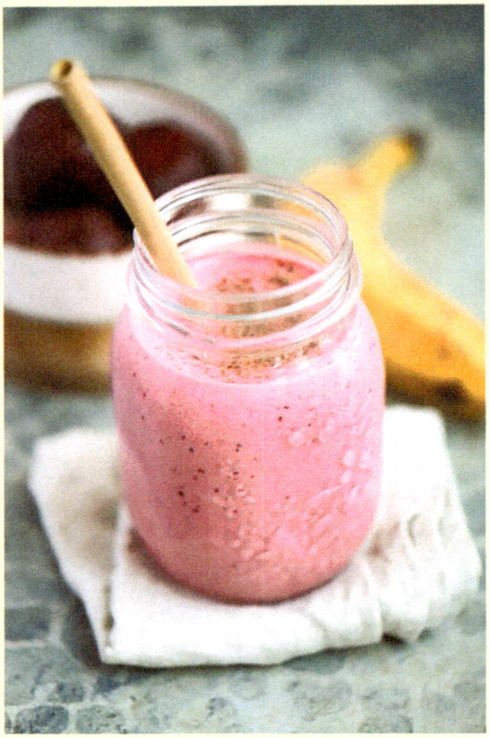
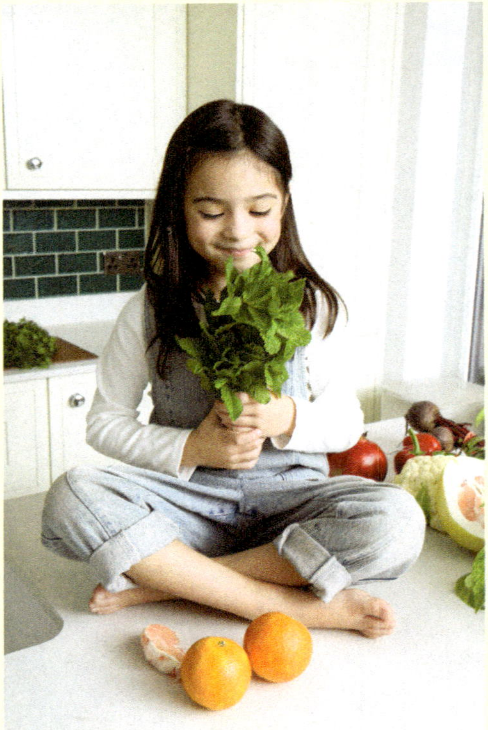

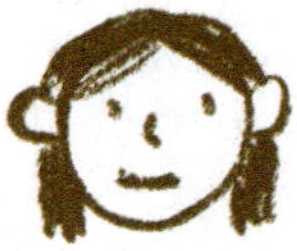

Overcoming Resistance from Family Members

It's Tuesday evening; I'm standing in the kitchen, surveying my latest culinary creation - a beautiful array of roasted vegetables that took me ages to prepare. I'm feeling pretty proud of myself until I see those all-too-familiar sceptical looks around the dinner table. Pia's eyeing the broccoli like it might jump off her plate and attack her, and I can feel my carefully planned healthy dinner turning into yet another mealtime challenge.

The Great Food Evolution

The other day, I was making a lovely chickpea curry for dinner, and it hit me - I used to be exactly like Pia! I vividly remember sitting at my parents' kitchen table, aged about seven, staring down at a plate of curry my mum had made. I was convinced that curry was disgusting and could not understand why people enjoyed it. The smell alone made me want to gag. Now, I absolutely love curry, and it's one of my go-to comfort foods. It really made me think about how our tastes change and evolve over time.

This revelation came in particularly handy last week when Pia was having a "broccoli breakdown." Instead of getting frustrated, I shared my curry story with her. "You know what, darling? Mummy used to hate curry, and now it's one of my favourite foods!" Her response? "So... one day, I might like broccoli?" Well, yes! However, she did follow that up with, "But not today, right?" Baby steps!

Team Health: The Family Project

Something I've learned both as a nutritionist and as a mum is that trying to be the food police doesn't work. Trust me, I've tried! The moment I started treating our health journey as a family project rather than "Mummy's crazy new idea" (an actual quote from Pia), everything changed.

Did you know the average UK family consumes nearly three times the recommended daily sugar intake? When I first learned this, I was tempted to go full sugar-police mode. But instead, I turned it into a family challenge. I set a goal to reduce our sugar intake by around 20%, and we all agreed that it was a good idea.

My approach wasn't about going cold turkey and eliminating all sugary snacks. Instead, it started with making our own treats. Pia became our official "taste tester," rating our creations. Sure, some experiments were more successful than others (the courgette and beetroot brownies were an epic fail), but watching her get excited about creating healthier versions of her favourite snacks was worth every failed attempt.

The Fitness Files

Remember when exercise meant just playing outside until your mum called you in for dinner? These days, it feels like we need to schedule every minute of activity. Having Pia has taught me that kids naturally want to move; we just need to make it fun rather than feel like a chore.

Last month, I decided to do a quick home workout because I didn't have time to get to the gym. There I was, trying to get through the burpees, when Pia wandered in and decided this looked like fun. Before I knew it, my "quick workout" had turned into what she called "Pia's Dance Party Fitness Show." She added 'burps' to my burpees, twirls to my squats, and made me do star jumps while singing "Let It Go." It was not exactly what I had in mind, but it got us both moving. We laughed, and it was probably the most fun I've had exercising in ages!

Did you know that around 80% of children in the UK don't get enough exercise? That statistic is a real shocker and actually made me feel quite sad. However, instead of worrying about it, I've chosen to get creative with movement. We often have spontaneous dance parties after dinner and enjoy quick games of 'The Floor is Lava' between homework sessions. Pia especially loves our 'Animal Walk' up the stairs - climbing like a crab. While she critiques my technique, she always brings in the laughs!

Operation Everyone's Involved

Planning in our house started as a way to avoid the daily 'What's for dinner?'

drama, but it's become a bit of a family affair - most days, anyway! Every Sunday, we have what Pia likes to call our 'Food Team Meeting.' It's really just us sitting at the kitchen table with some colourful markers and a weekly planner, but the title makes it sound fancier.

Each family member gets to choose one dinner for the week, with the only rule being it has to include at least one vegetable. Pia often tries to argue that ketchup counts as a vegetable. Her first choice is often 'Rainbow pasta' - which is just normal pasta tossed with whatever colourful veggies I could find and some cheese. Would she have eaten those vegetables if I'd just put them on her plate? Probably not. But since it was 'her' dinner, she was genuinely excited about it!

The Art of Compromise

Compromising was probably my biggest learning curve as both a nutritionist and a mum. I used to think that because I knew about nutrition, I had to be strict about everything we ate. Spoiler alert: that approach backfired spectacularly.

One memorable evening was when I'd made this delicious lentil shepherd's pie. I'd spent ages hiding vegetables in it, making it look appetising, the whole works. Pia took one look at it and declared, "Mummy, this looks like mud pie, yuck." Instead of getting into a battle about it, I did something that shocked us both - I laughed and asked her how to improve it.

We ended up turning it into what she called "treasure pie" - basically the same dish, but with little pieces of cheese hidden throughout like "golden treasure." Was it technically 'less healthy' after using up all the cheese? Yes. Was it worth it to see her actually eating and enjoying a plate full of lentils and vegetables? Absolutely!

CLEMMIE'S Tip

Kid-Friendly Lentil Shepherd's Pie

Don't let the name fool you. This is just as hearty as the Lamb version, and surprisingly popular, especially if you just call it Shepherd's Pie!

Check our recipes on our YouTube channel or scan the QR code

Celebrating the Wins - Even the Tiny Ones

Last Tuesday, Pia tried a single edamame bean—one tiny bean. We celebrated it like she'd just won an Olympic medal because sometimes, that one edamame bean is a bigger victory than an adult trying a whole new cuisine. We now have a 'try it Tuesday' tradition, which seems to be working well!

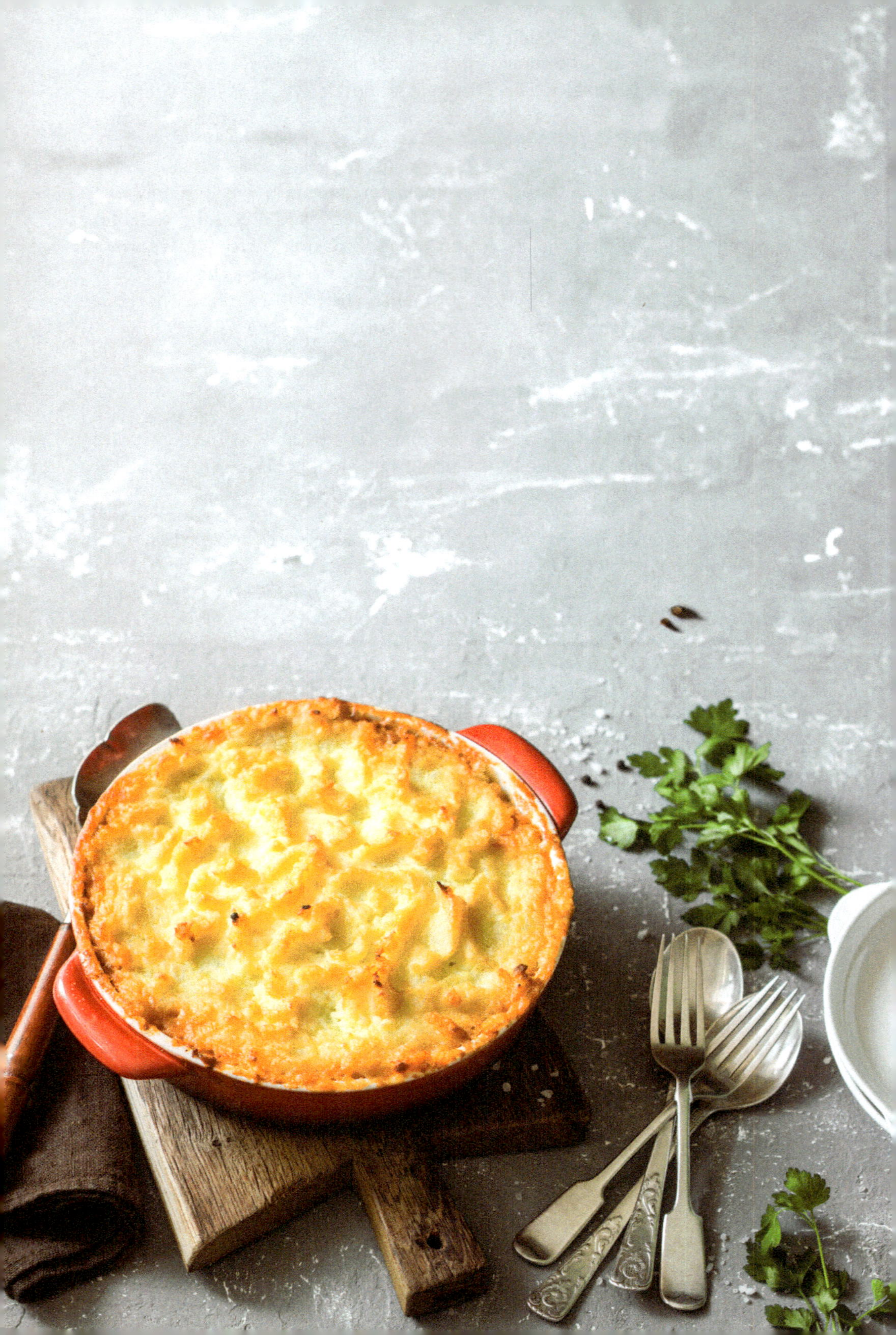

SHEPHERDS LENTIL PIE

Prep: 20 Min Cook: 40 Mins Total time: 1 hour

This is always a favourite and is a great one to make in bulk and freeze.

Serves 6

Filling:

1 tablespoon olive oil

1 small onion, finely chopped

1 carrot, diced small

1 celery stalk, diced small

1 courgette, grated

2 garlic cloves, minced

1 cup dried green or brown lentils, rinsed

1 can (400g) diced tomatoes

2 cups vegetable broth

1 tablespoon tomato paste

1 teaspoon dried oregano

1 teaspoon dried thyme

Salt and pepper to taste

Topping:

3-4 medium potatoes, peeled and cubed

1 tablespoon butter (or olive oil for a vegan option)

1/3 cup milk (or plant-based milk for a vegan option)

Salt to taste

Optional: a sprinkle of grated (or chunks!) of cheese on top for the 'hidden treasure'.

Instructions

Preheat your oven to 180˚C (350˚F).

In a pot, boil the potatoes until tender, about 15 minutes. Drain, then mash with butter, milk, and salt until smooth. Set aside.

Heat olive oil in a large pan over medium heat. Sauté the onion, carrot, and celery for about 5 minutes, until softened.

Add the grated courgette and garlic, and cook for an additional 2 minutes.

Stir in the lentils, diced tomatoes, vegetable broth, tomato paste, oregano, and thyme. Bring to a simmer, then cover and cook for about 20-25 minutes, or until the lentils are tender and the mixture thickens. Season with salt and pepper to taste.

Pour the lentil mixture into a baking dish.

Spread the mashed potatoes over the lentil mixture, smoothing with a spatula. If desired, sprinkle a small amount of grated cheese on top.

Place the dish in the oven and bake for 15-20 minutes, or until the top is golden and bubbly.

Let the pie cool for a few minutes before serving. Serve with a side of steamed veggies or a salad for extra nutrition!

CLEMMIE'S Tip

You can add a dash of paprika or mild spices to the potatoes for extra flavour.

Try calling it "shepherd's pie" to make it feel more familiar, or even add a little story about the "lentil shepherds" to make it fun!

We have this little chart in our kitchen fridge that we call our "Food Challenge Chart" (though really, it's just a corner of the fridge covered in Post-it notes and scribbles). Every time someone tries something new or makes a healthy choice, it goes up on the wall. Pia drew a picture of herself as a "bean-tasting superhero" after the great edamame bean incident, and one morning, I found Pia showing my partner her food chart because she'd chosen fruit instead of chocolate buttons for her after-school snack the day before. "Look, I made a healthy choice ALL BY MYSELF!" she announced proudly. Was I hiding around the corner, getting a bit emotional? Maybe. Did I also notice her sneaking an extra chocolate button after dinner? Yes. But that's okay, too - because this journey isn't about perfection but progress.

The Communication Game

Here's something they don't teach you in nutrition school – sometimes, the most important skill isn't knowing about vitamins and minerals; it's knowing how to listen. Really listen. It's not the "mm-hmm, that's lovely darling" kind of listening we all do sometimes when we're trying to cook dinner, get a wash on, and help with homework simultaneously.

Last month, Pia dropped this bomb at dinner: "Mummy, Sarah at school says carbs are bad for you." Instead of launching into my usual nutritionist spiel about complex carbohydrates and energy needs (trust me, I was tempted), I asked her what she thought about that. What followed was this amazing conversation about how different foods make us feel and how her body feels after eating different things. She even came up with this brilliant analogy about how cars need different types of fuel - and somehow decided that pasta was "supercharged rocket fuel" (I'm not correcting her on that one!).

The Reality Check

Let's have a really honest moment here - some days, despite all my knowledge and good intentions; dinner is fish fingers and frozen peas. And you know what? That's absolutely okay! I used to feel so guilty about this, like I was failing as both a nutritionist and a mother. But I've learned that health isn't always being perfect; it's about doing our best most of the time. My good friend Jade and I have a long-standing tradition we call "School Dinner Fridays" with her son Rex, one of Pia's best friends. Every other Friday (or whenever we can make it work), they come over, and I make the kids simple favourites like fish fingers, sausages, or pizza. Meanwhile, Jade and I unwind with a glass of wine and have a much needed catch up. This cosy ritual has been a staple for nearly five years now!

The other day, Pia caught me eating chocolate behind my laptop during a work call. Instead of trying to hide it (she has some kind of sixth sense for chocolate, I swear), I used it as an opportunity to talk about balance. "Yes, Mummy's eating chocolate," I told her. "Because sometimes we eat for nutrition, and sometimes we eat for joy, and both are okay."

What To Do Next

- Start your own "Food Challenge Chart"—grab some post-it notes and celebrate every tiny win. You can download our template for fun victory certificates from my website.
- Plan your first "Food Team Meeting" - make it fun with coloured markers and stickers. Let everyone choose one meal for the week ahead.
- Encourage movement throughout your day - have a set time, like after dinner, to pop a song on and dance, or if it's still light outside, pop out for an evening stroll before bath time.
- Try the "one bite, no pressure" rule. Create a star chart to track your new food adventures and use your smartphone to capture so of those priceless grimaces
- Start a family health journal. Let everyone contribute their thoughts and feelings about the food and activity choices you're making together.
- Plan your first "Try It Tuesday" - keep it simple and fun. Remember, even one pea counts as a victory! Make sure to keep it light-hearted and positive those first few times.
- Create your family's healthy living mission statement. Make it positive and achievable. Post it somewhere everyone can see it.
- Join the dedicated Facebook group, for readers of this book where parents share their food hero stories and creative ideas. Sometimes, the best inspiration comes from other parents in the trenches!

Chapter Nine

Instilling Lifelong Healthy Habits

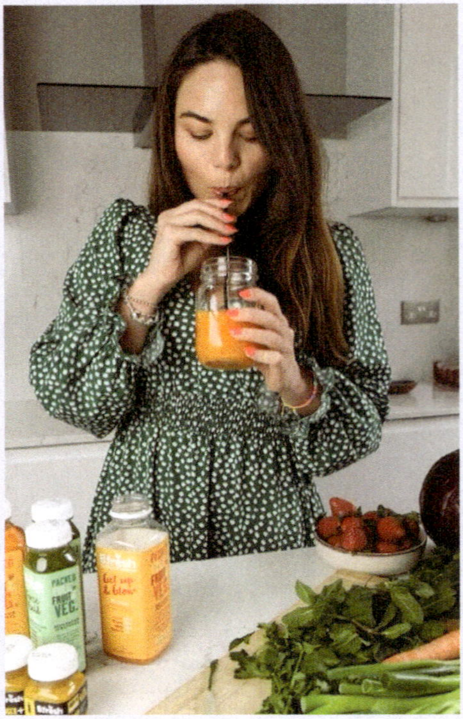
PACKED
FRUIT VEG.
Get up & blow

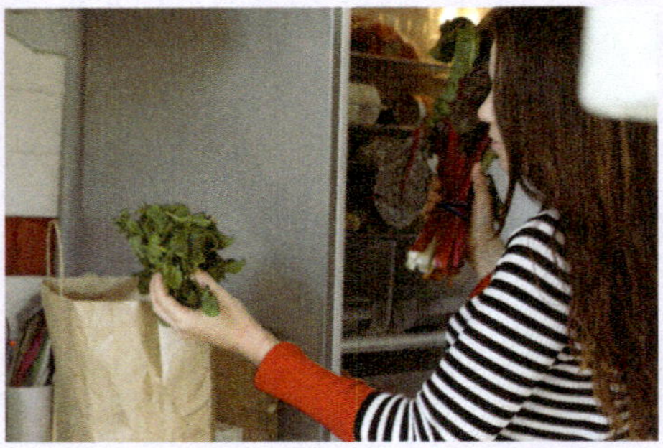

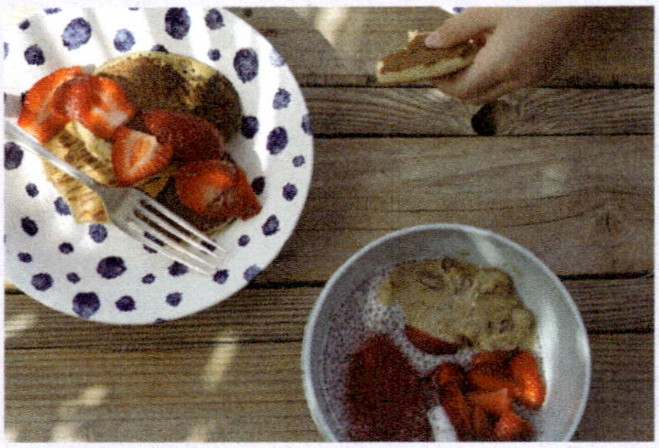

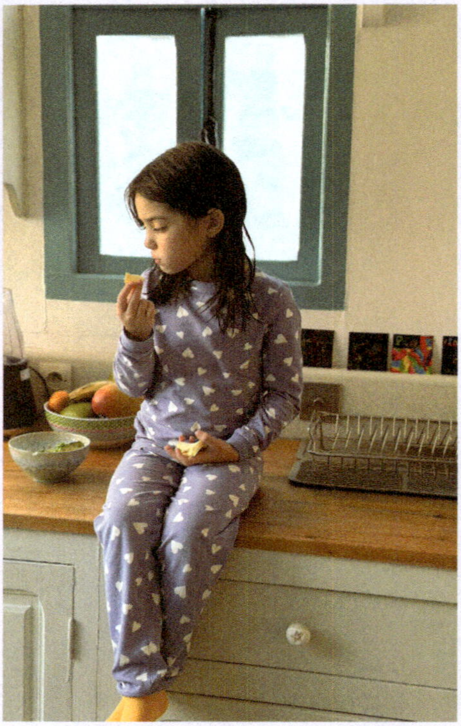

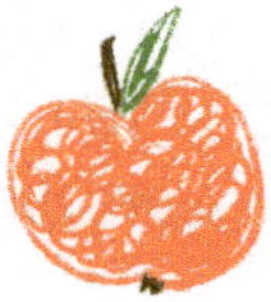

Instilling Lifelong Healthy Habits

You know those moments when you catch yourself saying something your mother used to say, and you can't quite believe it's coming out of your mouth? The other day, I heard myself telling Pia to "chew properly!" and had the most vivid flashback of my grandmother saying the same thing to me. There I was, standing in our kitchen, channelling generations of mums who've tried to get their kids to slow down and actually taste their food!

The Mindful Eating Journey

Our first attempt at mindful eating was both amusing and eye-opening. I'd set up this beautiful, calm dinner environment. Soft music was playing, candles lit (safely away from Pia's reach, obviously), and I'd planned to guide us through this lovely mindful eating exercise. Then reality hit. Pia was so excited about being "extra special quiet" that she whisper-shouted through the entire meal and somehow managed to turn her mindful breathing into a competition with herself about who could make the loudest "om" sound!

Even though it wasn't the serene experience I'd imagined, something magical happened. In all her enthusiastic whisper-shouting, Pia started noticing things about her food. "Mummy, did you know that broccoli looks like tiny trees? And if you look really close, they have little bumpy bits!" It wasn't quite the mindful eating exercise I'd planned, but she was paying attention to her food in a whole new way.

Ultra-Processed Food Reality Check

Before we dive deeper into mindful eating, I need to share something that terrifies me. Did you know that the UK has the highest number of children under seven needing general anaesthesia for tooth removal? When I first read that statistic, I nearly choked on my coffee. Children losing their baby teeth due to decay isn't just a dental problem; it's a glaring warning about our food environment. We're raising a generation that's lost touch with real food, and the repercussions go far beyond cavities.

Take this statistic: nearly 28% of children in the UK between the ages of 2 and 15 are classified as overweight or obese. Obesity rates have skyrocketed in recent decades, a trend that directly correlates with the rise in ultra-processed foods—foods packed with refined sugars, additives, and preservatives designed to make us crave more. These foods are engineered for taste, texture, and addictive quality rather than nutrition, which is why they're often irresistibly appealing to children. These "empty calories" aren't just an issue in the short term; they're paving the way for a lifetime of health challenges, including type 2 diabetes, heart disease, and even certain cancers.

It's scary to think about, but the convenience of processed food has come at the cost of health. In 2023, a report found that the average UK child consumes almost three times the recommended amount of sugar daily, most of it hidden in seemingly "harmless" packaged snacks, breakfast cereals, and even savoury items like bread and pasta sauce. These excess sugars, coupled with high levels of sodium and saturated fats in processed foods, put children at higher risk for metabolic syndromes, liver disease, and blood pressure issues. Processed foods are often stripped of natural nutrients, like fibre and essential vitamins, which can leave kids deficient in the very building blocks their growing bodies need. What's worse, processed foods are linked to behavioural issues, hyperactivity, and poor focus—all things that impact a child's development in school and social settings.

I remember the day Pia came home from school and proudly announced she'd swapped her oat cakes for a packet of fluorescent-coloured sweets. "But Mummy, they turn your tongue blue!" she excitedly informed me. It was such a striking reminder of how much of kids' social lives revolve around food. I know it would have been easy to launch into a lecture about artificial colours, preservatives, and sugar overload (believe me, I was tempted!). But I didn't want her to associate food conversations with shame or lectures; instead, I wanted her to feel curious about what she was putting in her body. So, we turned it into a little experiment. We made our own naturally coloured treats using beetroot powder and spirulina. Yes, the kitchen looked like a purple rainbow had exploded, and no, our tongues didn't turn quite as blue. But it opened up a fantastic conversation about how real food can be as exciting and colourful as processed stuff.

And that's the thing—real food doesn't need to be boring! When children experience the tastes, textures, and colours that come from nature, they're far more likely to develop a palate for nutritious foods. Studies show that children who are exposed to a variety of natural foods from a young age are less likely to develop picky eating habits and are more inclined to reach for fruits and vegetables as they grow older.

But the reality is that we're up against a well-oiled marketing machine. Processed foods are aggressively marketed to children, with colourful packaging, cartoon characters, and catchy slogans. A staggering 91% of adverts for food and drinks that target children in the UK are for products high in fat, sugar, or salt. These companies spend billions to keep their brands top of mind, often presenting their products as 'fun' and 'cool,' which makes natural food seem like a boring alternative. Choosing an apple over a sugary snack bar is almost a radical act for children.

Processed foods have become so normalised that eating whole, unprocessed foods feels like a departure from the norm. This shift in our food environment has also contributed to a rising incidence of nutrient deficiencies, with around 20% of British children found to be deficient in vitamin D, an essential nutrient for bone health and immune function. And it's not just vitamins and minerals; our reliance on refined grains and sugars over fibre-rich foods has led to a concerning rise in digestive issues, even among young children. Constipation, for example, is increasingly common in children who consume diets low in fibre and high in processed foods.

If I can share one thing I've learned from navigating these challenges with Pia, it's that kids are incredibly open-minded when we give them the chance to explore and experiment with real food. When they understand where their food comes from when they can taste, smell, and even play with it, they begin to see it as more than just fuel. For Pia, our homemade, naturally coloured treats weren't just food—they were an adventure. We talked about why we were using beetroots and spirulina, what natural pigments are, and how food can come in all sorts of beautiful colours without needing chemicals. She still reaches for sweets now and then, but she's also learning to appreciate the satisfaction that comes from eating something homemade, nutritious, and, yes, a little messy.

So, as we dive into the topic of mindful eating, let's remember: it's not about banning all processed foods or making children feel inadequate about their choices. It's about helping them reconnect with the joy of real, unprocessed foods, empowering them with knowledge, and creating memories around food that will last a lifetime.

Here are three practical tips on how to talk to kids about processed foods and help them build a positive, curious relationship with real food:

CLEMMIE'S *Tip*

Make It an Adventure, Not a Lecture: Rather than listing what's "bad" about processed foods, turn it into a learning adventure! Ask them if they know what's in their food, and let them explore labels and ingredients with you. Explain how certain ingredients, like added sugars and artificial colours, are used in processed foods to make them super appealing. You could even make a game of it, like asking them to count the ingredients on a snack label versus a piece of fruit.

Example: "Did you know apples have just one ingredient? Let's see how many ingredients are in this snack!"

CLEMMIE'S *Tip*

Get Hands-On with Real Food: Engage kids in making their own "fun food" with natural colours and flavours, just as you did with beetroot and spirulina. Show them how to make bright colours with fruits, vegetables, or spices, and let them help create their own snacks. This makes real food feel just as fun and exciting as the colourful processed snacks they see in stores.

Example: "What colour do you think these blueberries will turn your smoothie? Let's find out!"

CLEMMIE'S *Tip*

Focus on the Benefits, Not the Bans: Rather than saying, "Don't eat that," focus on the benefits of whole foods. Explain in simple terms how certain foods can help them feel stronger, run faster, or help their brains work better. This positive approach keeps the conversation light and empowering rather than restrictive.

Example: "Did you know carrots help keep our eyes sharp? Let's add some to our salad and see how they taste!"

These conversations make food a topic of curiosity and positivity, which helps children form their own understanding of healthy choices in a fun, engaging way.

The Routine Revolution

Let me paint you a picture of what our mornings used to look like: me frantically trying to pack a lunch while simultaneously attempting to convince a very sleepy Pia that, yes, she does need to put on both socks, not just one. It was chaos. Pure, stressful chaos.

Then, we discovered the power of routine, and while I can't say our mornings are perfect (I'm still finding random socks in strange places), they're more manageable.

We started what Pia calls our "Morning Mission," which is basically a routine. Everything sounds more exciting when you call it a mission, right?

Here's what happened when we first tried to establish our morning routine:

6:30 AM: Alarm goes off (in theory)

6:45 AM: Drag myself out of bed

7:00 AM: Attempt to wake Pia (this is where things used to go sideways)

But here's where we got creative. Instead of just trying to force a routine, we made it into a game. Pia now has her "Mission Morning Checklist," with little boxes to tick off: wake up like a superhero, power breakfast, pack lunch like a ninja, etc. It sounds silly, but it works! Most importantly, it's helped us establish consistent meal times, which is crucial for developing healthy eating habits.

On busy weeks, I often wake up an hour (or two!) before Pia. The calm and quiet of the early morning creates the perfect space for deep, focused work, journaling, or reading, and I notice my stress levels drop significantly. When I take the time to plan my mornings, I'm even more productive throughout the day. This routine may not be for everyone, but it sets me up for success, allowing me to accomplish way more with less overwhelm.

The Snack Strategy

Speaking of routines, I'd love to share our favourite healthy snacks that have become part of our daily rhythm. These aren't just random recipes - they're tested and approved by my very particular seven-year-old food critic:

CLEMMIE'S *Tip*

DIY Apple Sandwiches: Pia loves getting hands-on, so apple "sandwiches" have become one of our favourites! I slice an apple into thin rounds, spread peanut butter between two slices, and add fun fillings like raisins or granola for a little crunch. It's perfect because she feels like she's building her own snack, and I love how it's naturally sweet and packed with fibre. Plus, there's something so satisfying about watching her bite into these mini-sandwiches with that big apple crunch!

CLEMMIE'S *Tip*

Rainbow Veggie Cups with Hummus: For a while, Pia would only eat cucumbers and was suspicious of anything green! I started making "rainbow cups" by slicing different-coloured veggies—carrots, bell peppers, cherry tomatoes, and, of course, cucumbers and arranging them in small cups with hummus at the bottom. She loves the bright colours and getting to dip each veggie, and it's been a great way to get her excited about eating a variety of vegetables. Sometimes, we even make a game of it, guessing which colour she'll pick first!

CLEMMIE'S Tip

Frozen Yoghurt Bites: Pia has a sweet tooth, and I wanted to find a healthier option she'd still be excited about. We make frozen yoghurt bites by spooning a little Greek yoghurt into mini silicone moulds and adding bits of fruit - she loves blueberries and mango! After a few hours in the freezer, they turn into little yoghurt candies." She loves the icy texture, especially on warm days, and it's such a fun way to sneak in protein and probiotics. These are also great for snack bags if we're on the go.

CLEMMIE'S Tip

Banana & Nut Butter Roll-Ups: This one's a quick fix when we're in a rush but still want something filling. I spread a thin layer of almond or peanut butter on a whole wheat tortilla, place a banana in the centre, and roll it up like a burrito. It's one of Pia's favourites to help make, and we sometimes slice it into sweet "sushi" rolls for fun. It's a great way to get a little protein and healthy carbs, and it's perfect for taking along to after-school activities.

CLEMMIE'S Tip

Cheese & Fruit Kebabs: Pia loves anything that feels like an activity, so we started making "kebabs" with her favourite fruits and small cubes of cheese. We use thin, blunt-ended wooden skewers (safer for little hands!) and thread on grapes, apple slices, cheddar cubes, and strawberries. She loves choosing which fruit goes on next, and it's a fun way for her to mix and match flavours. I love that it combines protein and fresh fruit, making it both a filling and nutritious option. Plus, it's a great way to turn snack time into a mini art project!

Creating Food Independence

The hardest part of teaching kids about food isn't really about the food—it's about letting go of control. Setting up Pia's "snack station" in a lower kitchen cabinet was both terrifying and liberating. Sure, she sometimes makes some interesting combinations (dried apricots dipped in hummus, anyone?), but she's learning to listen to her body and make her own choices. Let them experiment!

The Independence Experiment

Our latest adventure in food independence was giving Pia a chance to plan and help prepare an entire day's meals. Brave? Maybe. Her menu began with "rainbow toast" for breakfast - toast topped with about seventeen different ingredients arranged in colour order. For lunch, she designed an "explorer's picnic," where every item had to be "discovered" from a different part of the kitchen. And for dinner, she created a "princess power" feast, with everything somehow turned purple (thank you, beetroot!).

Was it messy? Absolutely. Did we try some unusual flavour combinations? Without a doubt. But watching her confidence bloom as she made choices about food was worth every sticky surface and purple-stained counter. She even put together her own little recipe book, complete with illustrations that barely resemble the real dishes..but her excitement was contagious!

The Reward System Reality

I used to be quite anti-reward. As a nutritionist, I worried about creating unhealthy associations with food. But then I had this lightbulb moment while watching Pia collect stickers at school for reading. She wasn't just reading for the stickers; she was genuinely enjoying the books, and the stickers made it more fun.

So, we created a "Food Explorer's Map." Instead of just ticking off new foods tried, Pia draws a little picture of each new food and adds it to different "continents" on her map. Vegetables go in the "Green Kingdom," fruits in the "Sweet Islands," and so on. The reward isn't food - it's completing different "regions" of her map and earning special explorer badges (which are really just badges I found on Amazon, but don't tell her that!).

Making It All Work

Here's something I think we need to talk about - balance. Real, messy, imperfect balance. Last week, we had one of those days where everything went wrong. The morning routine fell apart; I had back-to-back work calls, and by dinner time, I was exhausted. Know what we had? Beans on toast. And you know what? That's okay, too.

I remember feeling guilty about it until Pia said something that stopped me in my tracks. Arranging her beans in a smiley face pattern, she said, "Mummy, we're still eating mindfully because I'm making my food happy!" It was so sweet!

Through my professional training and parenting adventures, I've learned that creating healthy habits isn't about perfection but consistency in our imperfections. It's about picking ourselves up after chaotic days and starting fresh the next morning.

Last night, I found Pia "reading" her Food Explorer map to her stuffed animals, telling them about the "brave princess pea" living in the Green Kingdom. She was making up this elaborate story about how the pea had special powers because it was so small but mighty. And, at that moment, I realised that all these little things we do - the mindful eating games, the silly routines, the explorer maps - are not just about nutrition. They're about creating a positive relationship with food that will hopefully last a lifetime.

Creating lifelong healthy habits isn't just about the food on the plate - it's about the joy, curiosity, and connection we create around that food. Sometimes, it's messy; sometimes, it's chaotic, but it's always worth it. And if you find yourself saying things your grandmother used to say about chewing properly, know that you're not alone. We're all in this together, one mindful bite at a time.

What To Do Next

1. Create your own Food Explorer's Map - download our template and let your kids decorate their food continents. Watch our video for creative ideas!
2. Set up a simple mindful eating practice - start with just one meal a day, where everyone takes three deep breaths before eating. Keep it light and fun!
3. Establish your own "Morning Mission" routine. Create a checklist template and customise it for your family's needs. Try and involve your child in its creation- this way they have ownership of it
4. Create a "Snack Station" at kid height. Check out my Amazon Shop for suggested items that I think work and of course there is a full list of suppliers with discount codes in chapter 14.
5. Start a weekly "Food Adventure Time" where kids help plan and prepare one meal. Don't worry if the first few go wrong! it's all part of learning together.
6. Begin a family gratitude practice at meals - take turns sharing one thing you're thankful for, even if it's just "yummy toast!" This often works best at supper time, when they can reflect on the day

7 Set up your first mindful tasting experiment. Try our "raisin exercise" or create your own version with different fruits. It always getting them asking questions, so be ready!

8 Follow me on Instagram and YouTube to get inspiration for your family's food adventures and get support from other parents on the same journey.

Chapter Ten

Smart Shopping for Nutritional Success

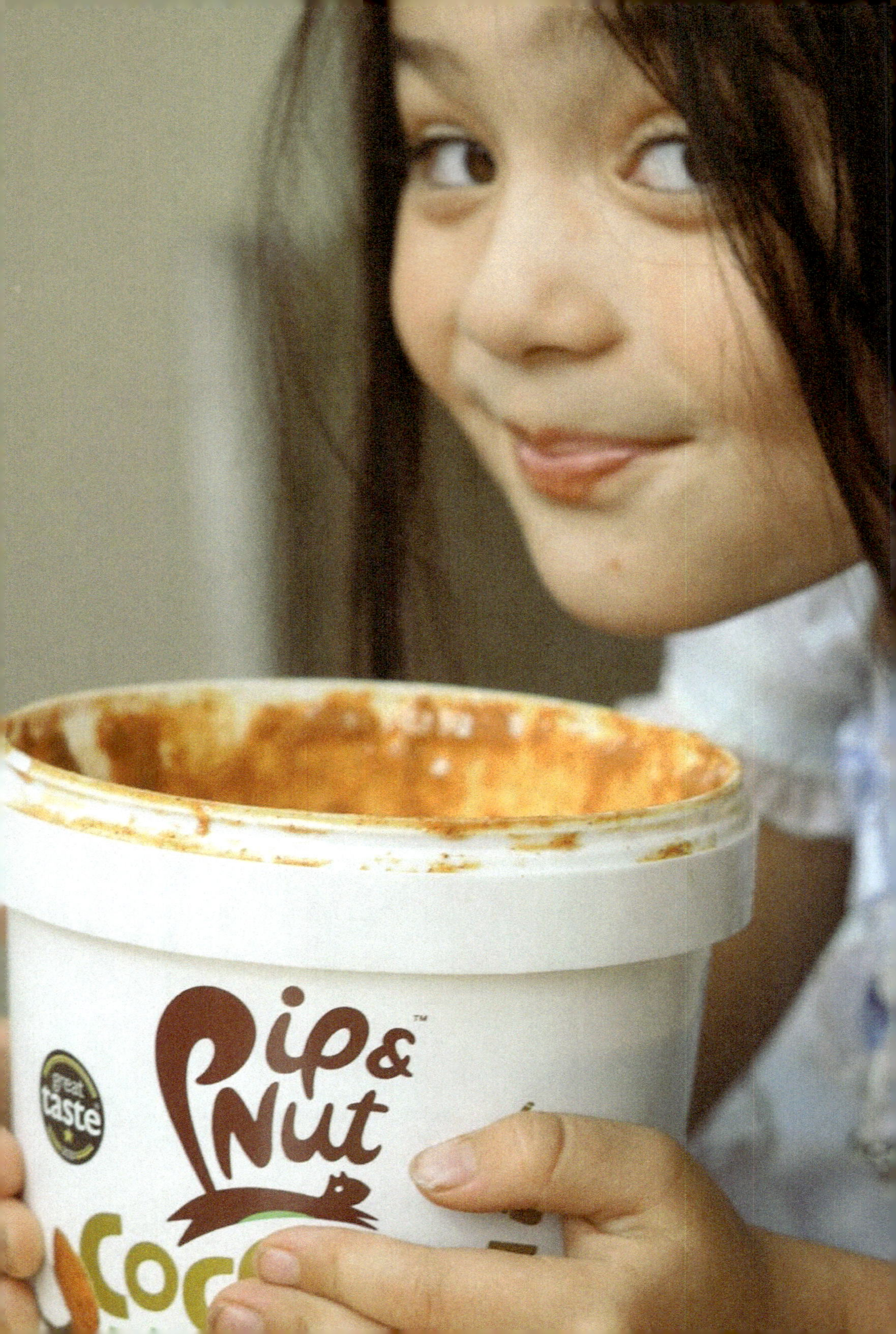
Pip & Nut
great taste

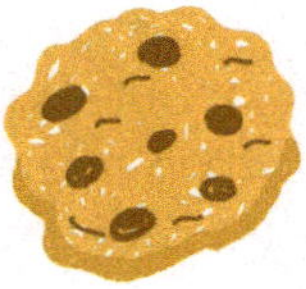

Smart Shopping for Nutritional Success

I'm standing in the middle of the supermarket, desperately trying to remember what I need for dinner while Pia's doing her best impression of a tornado in the cereal aisle. My shopping list is somewhere in my bag (probably covered in unicorn stickers), and I'm pretty sure I've walked past the same display of biscuits at least three times. Sound familiar? Trust me, I've been there more times than I care to count! But over the years, I've learned that turning these chaotic shopping trips into something more manageable isn't just possible - it can be enjoyable. Yes, really!

The other day, while I was attempting to navigate the produce section with Pia (who was determined to squeeze every single avocado), she asked me something that really made me think. "Mummy," she said, looking up at me with those big, brown eyes, "why do we always have to check our list?" It instantly transported me back to my own childhood, trailing behind my mum every Saturday morning at the supermarket. I remember how she'd methodically work through her carefully written list, checking off each item while I begged for something from the sweet aisle. Back then, I thought she was just being boring - now I realise she was actually teaching me one of the most valuable lessons about food shopping!

The Art of List-Making

Let's talk about shopping lists - and I know what you're thinking: "Really, Clemmie? A whole section about lists?" But stick with me here! The other morning, I was frantically searching through my bag at the supermarket checkout, only to find my carefully planned list had been transformed into Pia's latest art project. There I was, trying to remember what I needed while simultaneously stopping her from adding yet another packet of chocolate buttons to our trolley. We've all been there, right? That moment when you get home and realise you've forgotten the one thing you actually went shopping for!

That's precisely why I've become almost evangelical about shopping lists - and not just any lists, but ones that actually work for real life. Studies show that people who shop with lists save about 20% on their bills, which is amazing when you think about it. But here's the thing - it took me ages to figure out how to make lists that don't just end up crumpled in the bottom of my bag or completely ignored when those chocolate digestives start calling my name!

These days, I make lists during that precious window of time before Pia wakes up, when I'm nursing my coffee and can string two thoughts together. I've learned that taking fifteen minutes to plan things out saves hours of stress later. First, I think about our week ahead—is it a typical school week? Do we have any playdates coming up? Is there a birthday party where I need to bring something? All of these affect what needs to go on that list.

I used just to scribble down whatever came to mind, but now I plan our dinners for the week. Nothing fancy or complicated - we're talking simple, realistic meals that won't have me losing my mind at 6 PM while Pia's hanging off my leg asking for her third snack of the afternoon. I might jot down "Monday - hulk pasta (my nutrient-dense, green sauce that somehow still fools her) or "Wednesday - jacket potatoes" because I know we've got swimming lessons and need something quick.

The game-changer for me was when I started thinking beyond dinner. I now look at what we need for breakfasts, lunch boxes (which need to be interesting enough that they don't come home untouched), and snacks (because somehow, we go through an endless amount of rice cakes and fruit). I even check our "emergency supplies" - those things that save your sanity on tough days, like pasta and pesto or ingredients for quick quesadillas.

One of my best discoveries was moving my list to my phone – because let's face it, that's the one thing I never forget! I use a simple notes app, but there are loads of fancy shopping list apps out there if that's your thing. The real beauty of having it on my phone is that I can add things throughout the week as we run out. Pia's emptied the last of the milk? Straight on the list, it goes. Have I used up the last banana in her smoothie? On the list before I forget.

The Seasonal Shopping Adventure

It's mid-December, and I'm in the fruit aisle, trying to find decent strawberries. Pia was adamant she needed them for her breakfast, so I spent an embarrassing amount of time hunting through the produce section before finally finding some sad-looking strawberries that cost more than my morning coffee habit. That's when it hit me - fighting against the seasons is expensive and misses the point of fresh food.

During my nutrition training, we spent a lot of time learning about seasonal eating, but it wasn't until I started really paying attention to what was available that I understood why it matters so much. Those summer strawberries that burst with sweetness? They're nothing like their winter counterparts. And it's not just about taste - seasonal produce is usually cheaper (because there's plenty of it around), more nutritious (because it's been allowed to ripen naturally), and better for the environment, too.

I've turned seasonal shopping into a bit of an adventure with Pia. Spring brings us tender peas that she'll eat straight from the pod (a minor miracle in itself) and asparagus that we pretend are magic wands before cooking. Summer explodes with berries, tomatoes that actually taste like tomatoes (remember those watery winter ones?), and more courgettes than I know what to do with - though my famous chocolate and courgette cake usually helps use them up!

Autumn is our favourite season for comfort food shopping. We hunt for the perfect pumpkin, not just for Halloween but also for soup. The sweet potatoes and apples at this time of year are incredible, and I've learned to embrace their abundance by batch cooking and freezing. Winter might seem less exciting, but that's when our citrus fruits shine and all those hearty root vegetables come into their own. Even kale (which Pia still eyes suspiciously) tastes sweeter after a frost.

The Leftover Revolution

Can we have an honest conversation about leftovers? I used to be absolutely terrible with them. I'd find suspicious containers hiding at the back of the fridge, bearing little resemblance to their original contents—money literally in the bin! It wasn't until I started really thinking about food waste (and watching my food budget disappear) that I realised I needed to change my approach. I'm now practically the queen of leftovers and am not even slightly embarrassed about it!

Last week, I made a roast chicken on Sunday, trying to channel my inner domestic goddess. That one chicken then turned into three completely different meals. Sunday was our traditional roast (even though Pia only ate the crispy skin and potatoes). Monday, the leftover meat went into the most fantastic chicken and sweetcorn noodle soup (Pia's current favourite because she can slurp the noodles). By Tuesday, the remaining bits were transformed into quesadillas with cheese and vegetables. Even the bones didn't go to waste - they made a fantastic stock that's now sitting in my freezer, ready for the next time I need it. Talk about making your money work harder!

Cooking more than you need on purpose is always a great idea. When I'm roasting vegetables for dinner (sweet potatoes, carrots, whatever's in season), I'll throw in an extra tray. Those extras are great for 'throw together' salads, quick side dishes, or even blitzed into soup. The key is having a plan for them before they end up forgotten in the fridge. It's not technically leftovers if you meant to make extra, right?

The freezer has become my secret weapon in this leftover revolution. Those extra portions of bolognese sauce? Straight into freezer bags in portions perfect for quick midweek dinners. Surplus roasted vegetables? They'll be amazing in a frittata next week. Even those brown bananas that Pia refuses to eat (because apparently, even a single brown spot makes them "yucky") get peeled and frozen for smoothies, nice cream, or banana bread. It's like having a pause button for food!

Making Shopping a Family Adventure

Remember those old supermarket sweep shows? Well, that's basically what shopping with kids can feel like - minus the prizes and much more negotiation about the overpriced kid's snacks! But fighting against chaos sometimes creates more stress than just embracing it and turning it into something fun. These days, our shopping trips have become less of a battle and more of an adventure (most days, anyway!).

Last week, Pia announced she wanted to be the "shopping boss." Instead of immediately saying no (which was my first instinct, I'll admit), I decided to roll with it. I gave her a small notebook and let her create her own little shopping list with pictures she drew of things we needed. Yes, it took longer. Yes, some of her drawings were rather... creative (apparently, broccoli looks precisely like ice cream in her world). But you know what? She was engaged, learning, and actually excited about buying vegetables. Small wins!

I've found that giving kids real responsibility during shopping trips makes such a difference. Pia now has specific jobs that are "hers" - finding the ripest bananas (we call her the banana expert), counting out exactly six apples, or being in charge of the shopping list (with supervision, obviously, or we'd end up with nothing but Petit Filous and chocolate buttons). Not only does this keep her occupied, but it's also teaching her valuable skills about food selection and budgeting without her even realising it.

The produce section has become our favourite learning spot. We play "rainbow shopping," trying to find fruits and vegetables in every colour. It's turned into this beautiful game where Pia gets excited about finding purple cabbage or orange peppers. Sometimes, she'll spot something unusual - like dragon fruit or star fruit - and we'll buy it just to try something new. These experiments often end up being more educational than delicious, but that's all part of the adventure.

Real Life in the Supermarket

Look, I need to be honest here - as much as I love sharing all these tips and strategies, some days, it all goes out the window. There are times when I'm tired, Pia's exhausted, and we end up buying fish fingers and frozen peas because that's all we can manage. And you know what? That's perfectly okay! Being a nutritionist doesn't mean I'm immune to real life, and being a mum definitely means accepting that sometimes good enough is, well, good enough.

I remember one particularly challenging shopping trip where Pia had a complete meltdown in the middle of the store because I wouldn't buy the flavoured yoghurt with the cartoon character on the box that was basically pure sugar. There I was, trying to explain why we don't need this yoghurt, which is basically dessert in disguise, while she was crying about how 'unfair it was and that I never let her have anything she wanted". At that moment, all my carefully planned nutritional wisdom went right out the window, and I just needed to get through the shop without losing my mind. I bought the flavoured yoghurt.

These real moments are important to share because they remind us that we're all human. I believe in the power of meal planning and nutritious eating, but I also believe in being gentle with ourselves. Sometimes, the perfectly planned shopping trip goes entirely off the rails. Sometimes, we cave and buy the chocolate buttons. Sometimes, we grab whatever's quickest because we're exhausted, and it's been one of those days.

Kitchen Staples and Quick Recipes

I have a "survival shelf" - containing those items that have saved dinner (and my sanity) more times than I can count. The other day, Pia's playdate ran late. I'd completely lost track of time, and suddenly, it was 5:30 with two hungry kids staring at me expectantly. But thanks to my well-stocked cupboards, I managed to throw together a pretty decent meal without resorting to ordering pizza. It's moments like these when having a good stock of kitchen staples really proves its worth!

My must-have cupboard items have evolved over the years, partly through trial and error and partly through discovering what Pia will actually eat. Whole wheat pasta is always on hand (though let's be honest, sometimes only the white pasta will do), along with brown rice, quinoa, and those microwaveable grain pouches that are worth their weight in gold on busy days. Tinned tomatoes are absolutely essential - I buy them in bulk when they're on offer because I know we'll always use them. The same goes for beans of all varieties. Pia's current favourite is butter beans, which she calls "giant beans" and likes to pretend they are tiny pillows. Hey, whatever works!

Speaking of beans, here is my favourite emergency dinner recipe that's saved us countless times. I call it our "Quick Bean and Cheese Quesadillas," though Pia has renamed them "Mexican Pizza Sandwiches" (marketing is everything when it comes to kids, right?). They're so simple that Pia can help make them, which automatically makes them taste better, in her opinion. All you need is tortillas (I always keep.

Quick Bean and Cheese Quesadillas (a.k.a. Mexican Pizza Sandwiches)

CLEMMIE'S Tip

These Quick Bean and Cheese Quesadillas are perfect for a busy weeknight dinner, and they're a fantastic way for kids to get involved in the kitchen. Plus, with the creative name "Mexican Pizza Sandwiches," they're sure to be a hit with everyone!

Check our recipes on our YouTube channel or scan the QR code.

Another lifesaver recipe that works brilliantly with cupboard staples is "Chewy Oatmeal Cookies" - because they're incredibly forgiving and adaptable. The base is just oats, nut butter, and honey or maple syrup. From there, you can add chocolate chips or Raisins. Pia loves making these because there's no real way to mess them up, and they're perfect for lunch boxes or after-school snacks.

Chewy Oatmeal Cookies

CLEMMIE'S Tip

The base is just oats, nut butter, and honey or maple syrup. From there, you can add chocolate chips or Raisins. Pia loves making these because there's no real way to mess them up, and they're perfect for lunch boxes or after-school snacks.

Check our recipes on our YouTube channel or scan the QR code.

These Chewy Oatmeal Cookies are not only easy to make, but they're also packed with goodness and perfect for lunch boxes or after-school snacks. Enjoy!

Your Shopping Success Plan

After years of trial and error (emphasis on the error part!), I've finally figured out what works for our family when it comes to food shopping. But it didn't happen overnight, and it definitely wasn't a straight path to success.

The biggest game-changer for me was realising that I needed different strategies for different types of shopping trips. The big weekly shop needs proper planning and, ideally, a time when Pia and I are well-rested and well-fed (hungry shopping is dangerous shopping!). I try to go right after school drop-off on Friday mornings - the shops are quieter, and I can think straight. For top-up shops during the week, I've learned to keep them super focused - get in, grab what we need, and get out before anyone has a meltdown (including me).

One strategy that's worked wonders is the "perimeter power walk." Most supermarkets are laid out with all the fresh stuff - produce, dairy, meat, bread - around the outer edges. So we tackle those areas first when we're still feeling fresh and motivated. The middle aisles, with all their processed temptations, come last when we've already got our healthy essentials sorted. Plus, by then, Pia's usually running out of steam, which means less time for her to spot all the colourful packaging calling her name!

I've also learned to be strategic about introducing new foods or trying to get Pia excited about healthy choices. The middle of a busy Saturday afternoon shop is NOT the time to try and convince her that kale chips are just as good as regular crisps (spoiler alert: she's not buying it). Instead, I might get her involved in picking out a new fruit to try when we're doing a quick morning shop and she's in a good mood. Small victories, right?

Getting Kids Excited About Smart Shopping

Watching how Pia's relationship with food shopping has evolved since I started talking to her about it properly. Last week, we were in the supermarket when she spotted some bright orange carrots with the green tops still on. "Mummy," she exclaimed, loud enough for the entire produce section to hear, "these ones still have their hair!" Instead of rushing past (which I sometimes still do when we're in a hurry), I took a moment to chat with her about how carrots grow. Before I knew

QUICK BEAN AND CHEESE QUESADILLAS (A.K.A. MEXICAN PIZZA SANDWICHES)

Prep: 5-10 Mins Cook: 6-8 Mins per Quesadilla

Total: Approximately 20-25 minutes

Serves 4

Tortillas: 4 large (flour or whole wheat, your choice)

Tinned Beans: 1 can (black beans, kidney beans, or pinto beans, drained and rinsed)

Cheese: 1 cup (grated; cheddar, mozzarella, or a blend)

Veggies: 1 cup (chopped; use whatever you have on hand, like bell peppers, spinach, onions, or corn)

Olive oil or butter: for frying

Seasonings (optional): 1 teaspoon cumin, 1 teaspoon garlic powder, salt, and pepper to taste

These Quick Bean and Cheese Quesadillas are perfect for a busy weeknight dinner, and they're a fantastic way for kids to get involved in the kitchen. Plus, with the creative name "Mexican Pizza Sandwiches," they're sure to be a hit with the whole family!

Instructions

Prep the Ingredients: In a mixing bowl, combine the drained beans, cheese, and chopped veggies. If you're using seasonings, add them in now and mix everything together.

Assemble the Quesadillas: Take one tortilla and spread a generous amount of the bean and cheese mixture on one half. Fold the other half over to create a half-moon shape. Repeat with the remaining tortillas and filling.

Cook the Quesadillas: Heat a large skillet over medium heat and add a little olive oil or butter.

Once hot, place a folded quesadilla in the skillet. Cook for about 2-3 minutes on each side or until golden brown and the cheese is melted.

Remove from the skillet and keep warm while you cook the remaining quesadillas.

Serve: Slice the quesadillas into wedges and serve warm with your favourite toppings, such as salsa, guacamole, or sour cream.

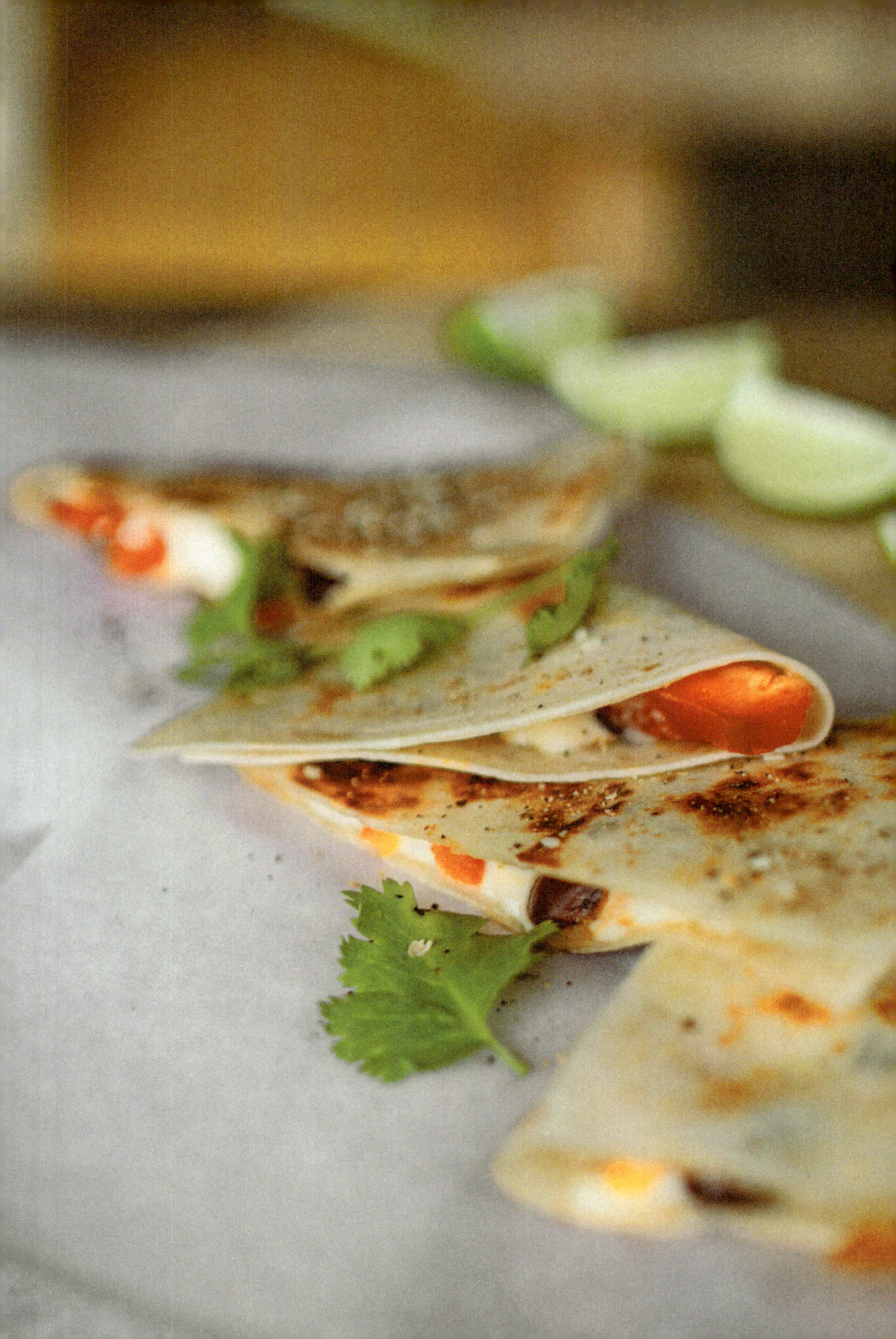

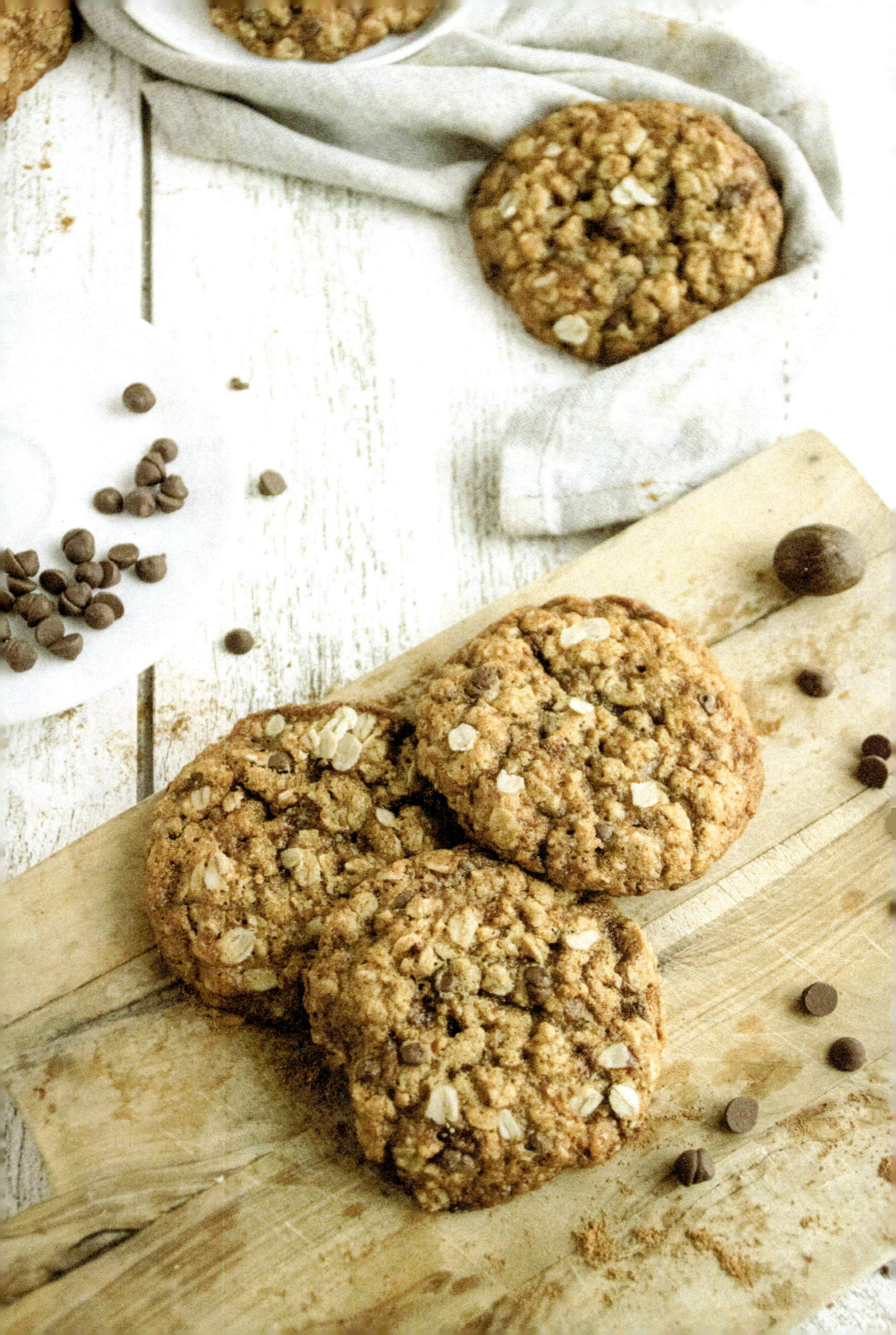

CHEWY OATMEAL COOKIES

Prep: 10 Mins   Bakek: 10-12 Mins

Total: 15-20 Mins

Makes 12-15

Oats: 2 cups (rolled oats work best)

Nut Butter: 1 cup (smooth peanut butter, almond butter, or any nut/seed butter you prefer)

Honey or Maple Syrup: 1/2 cup (adjust based on sweetness preference)

Chocolate Chips or Raisins: 1/2 cup (or a mix!)

Optional Add-ins (choose any combination):

1/2 cup chopped nuts (walnuts, almonds, or pecans)

1/4 cup seeds (chia seeds, flaxseeds, or pumpkin seeds)

1 teaspoon vanilla extract

1/2 teaspoon cinnamon

These Chewy Oatmeal Cookies are not only easy to make, but they're also packed with goodness and perfect for lunch boxes or after-school snacks. Enjoy!

Instructions

Preheat the Oven: Preheat your oven to 180°C (350°F) and line a baking tray with parchment paper.

Mix the Base Ingredients: In a large mixing bowl, combine the rolled oats, nut butter, and honey or maple syrup. If you're using vanilla extract and cinnamon, add them in now as well. Stir until everything is well combined.

Gently fold in your chocolate chips, raisins, and any other optional add-ins you've chosen.

Using a tablespoon, scoop out portions of the dough and place them onto the prepared baking tray. Flatten each cookie slightly with the back of the spoon or your hands, as they won't spread much during baking.

Bake in the preheated oven for 10-12 minutes or until the edges are lightly golden. Keep an eye on them, as they can go from perfect to over-baked quickly!

Remove the cookies from the oven and let them cool on the baking tray for a few minutes before transferring them to a wire rack to cool completely.

it, we were having this amazing conversation about vegetables coming from the ground, and she was genuinely excited about trying them. These little moments are pure gold.

I've discovered that turning shopping into a game changes everything. Remember those awful trips where every aisle felt like a battle? Now we play "Shopping Detective" - Pia has her own little notebook (decorated with unicorns, obviously) where she draws pictures of what we need to find. The other day, she spent ages looking for the "roundest orange" in the fruit section. Did it take longer than just grabbing the first orange I saw? Absolutely. But she was learning about choosing fresh fruit without even realising it, and she actually ate that orange as soon as we got out of the supermarket

One game that's become a favourite is our "Rainbow Challenge." We try to find fruits or vegetables in every colour of the rainbow. It started as a way to keep her entertained, but it's turned into this wonderful learning opportunity. Red tomatoes, orange peppers, yellow bananas - you get the idea. The purple ones always excite her - something about purple carrots or purple cauliflower just seems magical to her. And I've noticed she's more likely to try new foods when she's been involved in choosing them.

The money side of things has been fascinating to tackle. I'll never forget when Pia asked why we couldn't buy everything in the shop. Instead of just saying no, I gave her a £2 coin and told her she could choose whatever fruit she wanted within that budget. Watching her weigh up her options (quite literally with the bananas!) was amazing. She spent ages comparing prices and counting out pieces of fruit. In the end, she chose a punnet of strawberries over a bigger bag of apples because "they're more special." That little lesson in budgeting sparked so many great conversations about making choices with money.

These days, I give her small challenges, like finding the best value pack of her favourite crackers or comparing the prices of different brands. Sometimes, she'll spot that two smaller packs on offer are cheaper than the big pack - she's becoming quite the savvy shopper! It's not just about saving money; it's about helping her understand that our choices matter, both for our wallets and our health.

Speaking of health, I try to make the nutrition bit fun rather than preachy. Nobody wants a lecture in the middle of Tesco! Instead, we talk about "growing foods", "energy foods", and "brain foods." Pia now knows that fish is "brain food" because it "helps her think better at school," and she gets excited about choosing which one we'll have for dinner. When she asks why we can't have chocolate for breakfast (a regular question in our house!), we talk about how different foods make our bodies feel. She's starting to understand that while chocolate is lovely, it doesn't give her the same kind of energy as her dippy eggs.

The real magic happens when we get home, though. That's when all our shopping adventures come together in the kitchen. Pia has her own special apron (covered in unicorns, which matches her shopping notebook, of course), and she takes her role as sous chef very seriously. The other evening, we were making dinner together, and she told my partner all about how she'd chosen the "perfectly ripe" avocados for our salad. She was so proud! Even if she only ends up eating the grated carrot out of that salad, she's learning about food in such a natural, positive way.

Sometimes, our cooking sessions look like a flour bomb has gone off in the kitchen, and yes, things take about three times longer than if I had done them myself. But watching her face light up when she serves something she's helped make is worth all the mess in the world. Plus, I've noticed she's much more likely to try new foods when she's been involved in the whole process - from choosing them at the shop to helping prepare them at home.

The best part about all of this is not just teaching them about food - we're building memories and habits that will last a lifetime. I still remember helping my mum pick out peaches at the market, learning how to tell when they were perfectly ripe - those little moments shaped how I think about food today. Now, watching Pia develop her own relationship with food shopping and cooking, I realise we're creating her food memories, too. And yes, some days, we still have meltdowns in the biscuit aisle, but that's all part of the journey, right?

After all, isn't that what we really want? Not just kids who eat their vegetables but children who grow up understanding food, knowing how to shop smartly, and actually enjoying the whole process. I'm still working on convincing Pia that Brussels sprouts are exciting. Some battles are more challenging to win than others!

Looking Ahead

As I wrap up this chapter, I want to leave you with something I read recently that's stuck with me: "Shopping is where all your good intentions about healthy eating either come together or fall apart." At first, I thought it sounded a bit dramatic, but now I get it. Those choices we make in the supermarket shape our family's eating habits in such a fundamental way.

But here's what I really want you to remember: It's not about being perfect. It's about making small, manageable changes that work for your family. Maybe you'll start by making a proper shopping list, or perhaps you'll try involving your kids in the shopping process. Whatever you choose to try first, remember that every positive change, no matter how small, is a step in the right direction.

Next time you're standing in the supermarket, feeling overwhelmed (because, let's face it, we've all been there), take a deep breath and remember - you've got this. And if all else fails, eggs on toast is a perfectly acceptable dinner sometimes. Trust me, I'm a nutritionist!

What to Do Now

1. Create a Smart Shopping List: Before heading to the store, plan your meals for the week and write a detailed shopping list. This will help you stay focused and reduce impulse purchases.
2. Embrace Seasonal Eating: Research which fruits and vegetables are in season and incorporate them into your meals. This not only enhances flavour but can also save you money.
3. Get Creative with Leftovers: Turn leftover ingredients into new meals. For instance, repurpose last night's chicken into quesadillas or salads.
4. Stock Up on Superfoods: Include budget-friendly superfoods like beans, lentils, and oats in your grocery list. These are nutritious, versatile, and economical.
5. Use Technology for Savings: Download supermarket apps to access digital coupons and join loyalty programmes for exclusive discounts.
6. Check for Weekly Specials: Before shopping, look for ads in local newspapers or online to find discounts on items you frequently buy, including buy-1-get-1-free offers.
7. Shop in Bulk: Consider buying in bulk for non-perishable staples like pasta, rice, and canned goods. This can lead to significant savings over time.
8. Involve the Family: Create a smart shopping checklist together, encouraging kids to participate in the planning and shopping process. This can make it a fun family activity and instil good habits.

Chapter Eleven

Cultural Diversity in Family Meals

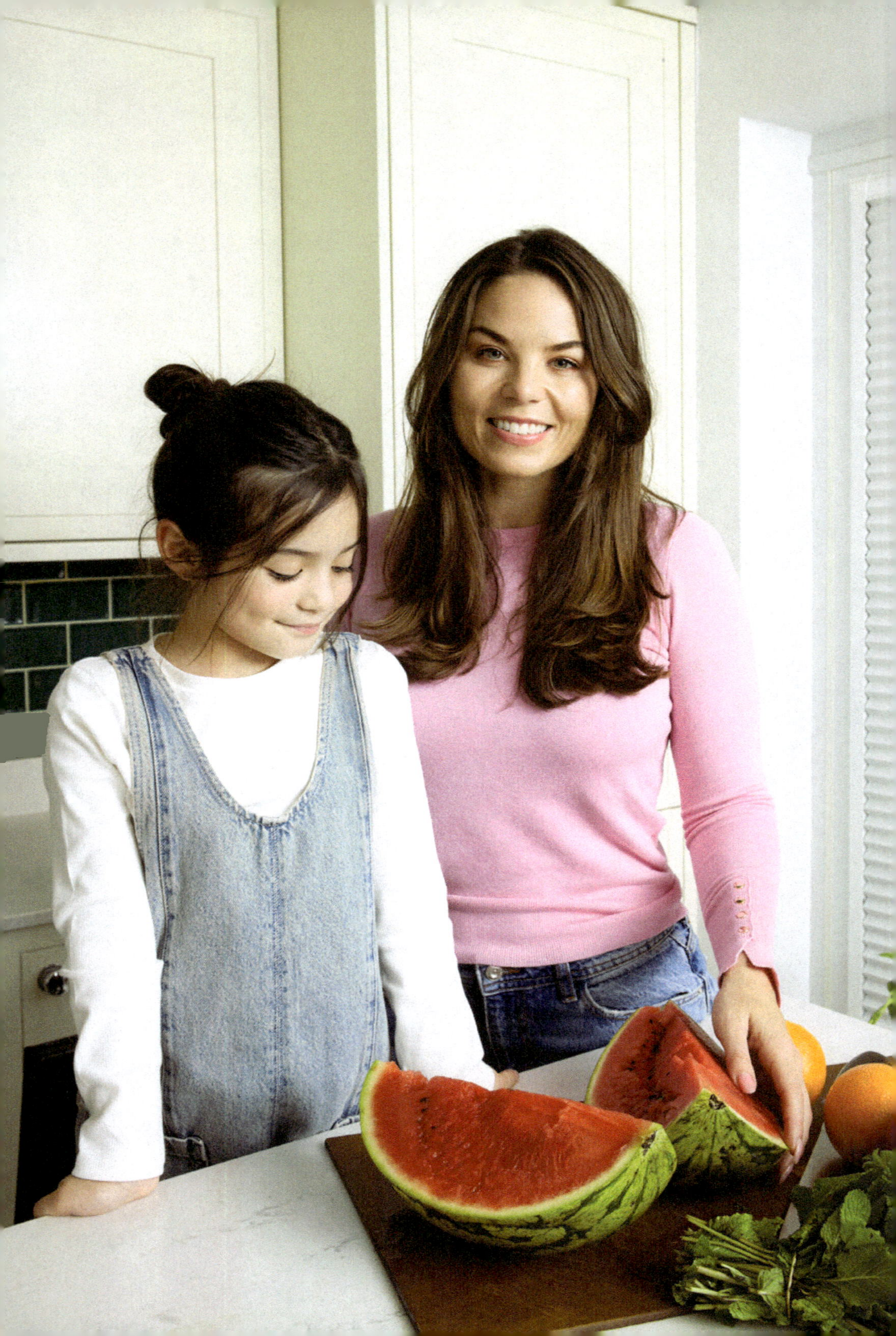

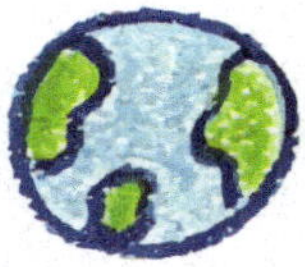

Cultural Diversity in Family Meals

I'm in the kitchen, attempting to fold dumpling wrappers (emphasis on 'attempting'), while Pia's sitting at the counter, totally engrossed in her dumpling-making mission. She might be making them look more like crushed fortune cookies, but her enthusiasm is off the charts! "Mummy," she asks, carefully crimping the edges of a particularly unique-looking dumpling, "did you know that in China, they eat these for good luck?" I'm not entirely sure where she picked up that fact, but watching her face light up as she shares this little piece of cultural knowledge makes my heart soar.

Moments like these remind me why exploring different cultures through food is so incredibly powerful. Here in London, we're surrounded by such fantastic diversity - did you know there are over 300 languages spoken in our city alone? That's 300 different cultures, each with their own beautiful food traditions just waiting to be discovered. And the best part? We get to explore all of this right from our own kitchen!

Embracing Your Culture

Pia is half-Colombian, or as she likes to call it, half "Latina," and I love embracing that part of her heritage - I'm also a little envious of her year-round, beautiful olive skin! I've always had a soft spot for Colombian food and have fond memories of living off buñuelos, those golden-brown deep-fried dough balls filled with cheese, during my pregnancy. I'm pretty sure I gained half the baby weight from those delicious little bombs. Now, Pia is just as obsessed with them as I am! It's so special to see her excitement when we talk about her Colombian roots. Maybe one day, we'll even take a trip to Colombia and experience the food and culture firsthand. But for now, we'll stick to the amazing Colombian restaurants in Elephant and Castle. They're definitely worth the trip!

It's important to embrace your culture and keep it alive for your children. Whether it's through food, language, or traditions, sharing your heritage with your kids can create lasting memories and a strong sense of identity. I'm so grateful for the opportunity to share this part of Pia's heritage with her, and I can't wait to see how she embraces her Colombian roots as she grows older.

Making Every Meal an Opportunity

You might think, "That's lovely, Clemmie, but my kids won't even eat regular pasta, let alone try foods from different cultures!" Trust me, I get it. Pia went through a phase where anything green was immediately suspicious, but I've learned that it's not about forcing kids to try everything; it's about making the exploration fun and natural.

The other day, we were having our usual breakfast when Pia asked why we always eat eggs in the morning. This turned into a sweet conversation about how different cultures start their day. We talked about how, in Japan, kids might have rice and miso soup for breakfast, and in Mexico, they might enjoy spicy eggs with tortillas. She was genuinely interested, and that curiosity was the first step.

I've found that starting with something familiar and adding a slight twist often works wonders. Take our "world tour of sandwiches" for example. We began with Pia's favourite cheese sandwich but gave it a cultural makeover each week. One week, it was a French croque monsieur (a fancy cheese toastie – an instant hit!); another week, we tried Vietnamese banh mi (she picked out the pickled vegetables but loved the crusty bread). Each sandwich came with a story about its origin, and slowly but surely, Pia started getting excited about trying new versions of familiar foods.

Making Global Foods Part of Your Regular Routine

Sometimes, the most profound changes happen almost by accident. I was desperately trying to break up the monotony of our weekly menu. I was so tired of hearing "pasta again?" (even though Pia would happily eat pasta seven days a week). Now, I'm trying to pick a different country's cuisine to explore each week.

Last Wednesday, we "visited" Thailand. Green curry is always a crowd-pleaser - for Pia, it was a very simple noodle stir-fry with a hint of Thai-inspired flavours. Pia helped me squeeze lime over everything (with slightly too much enthusiasm - our dinner was VERY citrusy), and we ate sitting on cushions on the floor because she'd learned that some Thai families eat this way. It probably wasn't the most authentic of Thai dinners but did it spark conversations about different eating customs and get her excited about trying new flavours.

Speaking of customs, we've started adopting different mealtime traditions from around the world. Pia's current favourite is saying "bon appétit" before meals. She picked it up from a cartoon and now insists we all say it, no matter what we're eating. This has led to some lovely conversations about gratitude and how different cultures express it. Her pronunciation is probably even better than mine!

Kid-Friendly Green Thai Curry

CLEMMIE'S *Tip*

Here's a mild, kid-friendly Green Thai Curry recipe that kids aged 4-8 will enjoy. It's flavorful but gentle on spice, and you can adjust the ingredients based on what your child prefers!

Check our recipes on our YouTube channel or scan the QR code.

CLEMMIE'S *Tip*

Here are some other fun tips to make the most of your Green Thai Curry:

Veggie Rainbows: Use different coloured veggies to create a rainbow in the curry!

Hands-on Creativity: Let kids use cookie cutters to shape the rice into stars or hearts for serving.

Personal Spice Levels: If they love adding flavours, let kids drizzle a bit of honey or pineapple juice to make it sweeter to their taste.

Sweet & Creamy Chickpea Curry

CLEMMIE'S *Tip*

This sweet, mild curry is sure to be a family favourite. It's quick to make, and the kids can really get involved in the preparation of the vegetables. It's almost as much fun making it as it is eating it!

Check our recipes on our YouTube channel or scan the QR code.

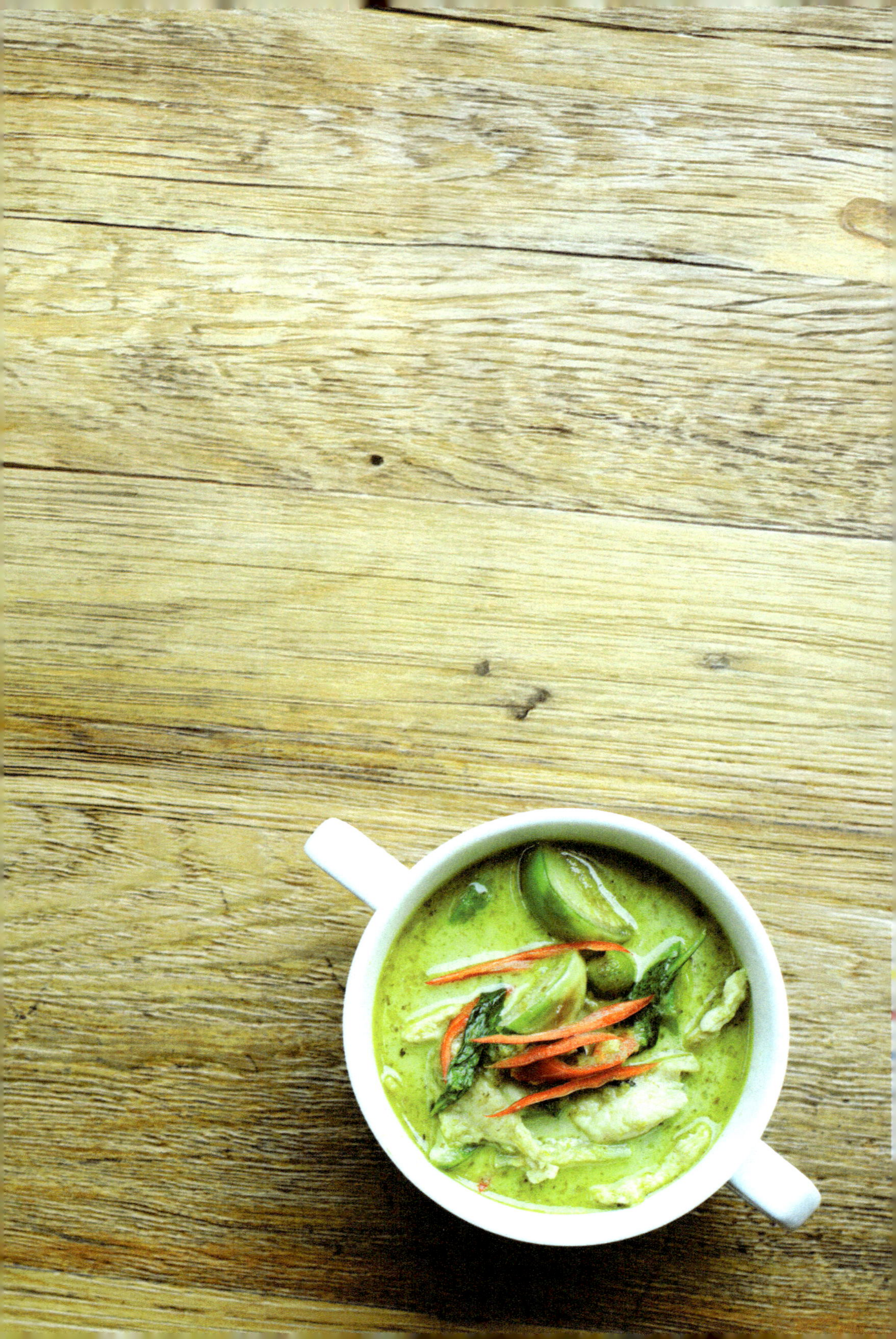

KID-FRIENDLY GREEN THAI CURRY

Serves 4

Prep: 30 Mins Cook: 5 Mins

Total: 35 Mins

Oats: 2 cups (rolled)

1 tbsp mild olive oil or coconut oil

1 small onion, finely chopped

1 clove garlic, minced

1 small piece of ginger (about 1 inch), grated

1 bell pepper (red or yellow), chopped

1 medium carrot, thinly sliced

1 small zucchini, chopped

1/2 cup broccoli florets (cut into small pieces)

1 cup coconut milk (use full-fat for creamier curry)

1 tbsp mild green curry paste (use less for a very mild taste)

1 cup vegetable or chicken broth

1 tsp brown sugar (optional, for mild sweetness)

1 tbsp soy sauce or coconut aminos

1/2 cup cooked chicken, tofu, or shrimp (optional for added protein)

Fresh lime wedges and a few basil leaves for garnish

Prep the Veggies (Kid's Job!):

Let kids wash the bell pepper, carrot, and zucchini.

For older kids, help chop the vegetables into small, bite-sized pieces. Younger kids can break apart the broccoli florets by hand into "mini-trees!"

Sauté the Aromatics (Grown-Up Step):

In a large pan, heat the oil over medium heat. Add the onion and cook until softened (about 3 minutes). Then add garlic and ginger, and stir for another minute until fragrant.

Add the Veggies (Kid's Job!):

With supervision, kids can toss in the bell pepper, carrot, courgette and broccoli. Have them help "stir the rainbow" for about 3-4 minutes until the veggies begin to soften.

Add Coconut Milk & Curry Paste (Fun Swirl for Kids!):

Pour in the coconut milk, green curry paste, broth, and brown sugar. Let kids use a spoon to stir and watch the curry paste swirl into the coconut milk—it's like making "green magic!"

Simmer & Add Protein (Grown-Up Step):

Let everything simmer for about 5 minutes to let the flavours blend. If you're adding cooked chicken, tofu, or shrimp, stir it in and cook for another 5-7 minutes until everything is heated.

Season the Curry (Taste Test Fun!):

Stir in soy sauce or coconut aminos. Let kids do a small "taste test" to see if they want a bit more sweetness or coconut milk for extra creaminess.

Serve (Kid's Job!):

Spoon the curry over rice or noodles. Kids can sprinkle basil leaves on top and add their own lime juice for a tangy twist.

SWEET & CREAMY CHICKPEA CURRY

Prep: 30 Mins

Serves 4

- 1 tbsp coconut oil or mild olive oil
- 1 small onion, finely chopped
- 1 clove garlic, minced
- 1/2 inch piece of ginger, grated (optional for a little flavour boost)
- 1 can (400g) chickpeas, drained and rinsed
- 1 medium carrot, finely diced
- 1 small sweet potato, peeled and diced into small cubes
- 1/2 bell pepper (red or yellow), diced
- 1 cup coconut milk (full-fat for extra creaminess)
- 1/2 cup vegetable or chicken broth
- 1 tbsp mild curry powder
- 1 tbsp honey or maple syrup (for a touch of sweetness)
- 1/2 tsp cinnamon (optional for added warmth)
- Salt to taste

Instructions

Get your mini-chefs to help! They can wash the carrot and sweet potato while you chop them into small pieces.

In a large pan, heat the coconut oil over medium heat. Add the onion and cook for about 3 minutes until it's soft. Add the garlic and ginger and cook for another minute.

Add the carrot, sweet potato, bell pepper, and chickpeas to the pan. Stir everything together for a couple of minutes.

Pour in the coconut milk and broth, then sprinkle in the curry powder, cinnamon (if using), and honey. Stir it all up and bring to a gentle simmer.

Let everything simmer for about 15 minutes until the vegetables are soft and the curry is creamy.

Add a pinch of salt and taste-test together. Let your child sprinkle on a little more cinnamon or honey if they like it sweeter!

Spoon the curry over rice or with naan bread on the side. For extra fun, let your little one sprinkle some fresh coriander on top.

CLEMMIE'S Tip

Make It Colourful: Use red or yellow bell peppers for a pop of colour!

Flavour Adventures: Encourage them to taste the curry along the way and describe the flavours.

Serve with Fun Sides: Try serving it with mini naan bread or even with a small side of apple slices for extra sweetness.

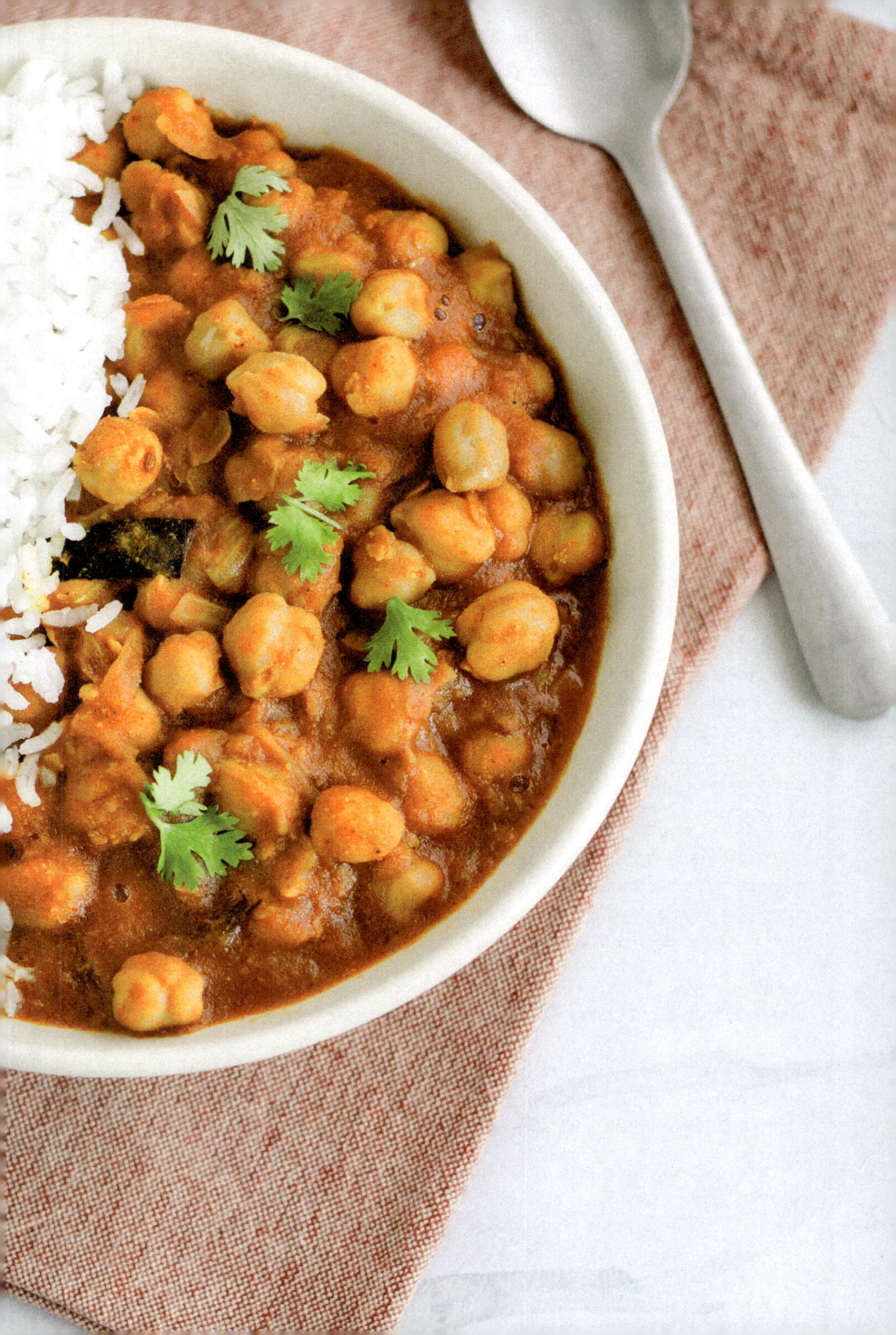

When Picky Eating Meets Cultural Exploration

Let's talk honestly about picky eating and cultural foods because this can be tricky territory! I remember feeling so frustrated when Pia wouldn't try the chickpea curry I'd made, even though I was so sure she would love chickpeas. But I've learned that sometimes it's about taking baby steps and finding creative ways to make new foods feel familiar.

One strategy that's worked brilliantly for us is making sure there's at least one element that I know Pia will eat. For example, when we tried Vietnamese summer rolls, I included cucumber (her favourite vegetable) alongside the more unfamiliar ingredients. She started by eating just the cucumber but gradually became curious about the other flavours, too.

Here's a perfect example: Our Indian food journey started with naan bread because what kid doesn't love bread? Once she was comfortable with that, we introduced very mild dahls, then rice dishes, and slowly worked our way up to more complex flavours. Now, she is a firm fan of mango lassis and even helps me make it!

Creating Your Own Global Kitchen

Our kitchen has slowly transformed into a "world market." The spice rack has expanded dramatically (though I still can't pronounce half the spices correctly), and our cupboards now house ingredients from all over the globe. Pia has her own special section where she keeps her "international ingredients" - currently consisting of nori sheets (for her unique sushi creations), Thai sweet chilli sauce (which she'd put on everything if I let her), and a collection of different kinds of rice that she likes to compare.

I've learned that it's not about having every authentic ingredient or making everything from scratch. Sometimes, we use shop-bought curry pastes or pre-made dumpling wrappers, and that's perfectly fine! The goal isn't to become master chefs of every cuisine - it's about opening our minds and palates to new experiences.

Building Lasting Cultural Appreciation

Last week, I had a very proud moment with Pia. She was talking about a snack her friend brought to school, and when another child called it "weird," Pia confidently replied, "It's not weird, just different—that's what makes food interesting.

These conversations about food have naturally led to broader discussions about culture, respect, and appreciation. Pia now understands that when we try foods from different cultures, we're not just eating – we're learning about people, traditions, and histories. She's becoming more mindful about using words like "gross" or "weird" when encountering new foods, instead asking questions about their origins and significance.

I encourage you to start your own cultural food journey. It doesn't have to be grand or perfectly executed. Maybe it starts with trying a new type of bread from your local bakery or picking up an ingredient you've never used before. The goal isn't to become experts in global cuisine – it's about fostering curiosity, respect, and openness to new experiences.

Remember, every family's journey will look different. Some kids might dive right in, eager to try everything, while others might need more time and gentle encouragement. What matters is creating an environment where different cultures are celebrated and exploration is encouraged.

In our house, we keep a little scrapbook in the kitchen called our 'Food Adventure Journal' that Pia uses to draw pictures of new dishes we try, writes down words she's learned from different cultures, and rates everything with her unique emoji system (apparently, Thai green curry gets three stars and a heart-eyed cat). It's becoming this wonderful record of culinary adventures, and I know it's something she'll treasure as she grows older.

Next time you're meal planning or food shopping, why not let your little ones choose a new country to explore? You might be surprised at where your taste buds take you! And remember, if your first attempt at making sushi looks more like a rice food fight (speaking from experience), that's all part of the adventure.

What to Do Next

1. Pick one new cuisine to try this week. Start with something simple, like Italian (if you've never made pizza from scratch) or Japanese (if your little ones like noodles). Check your cupboards for ingredients or add them to your shopping list.
2. Create your family's Food Adventure Journal. Grab a scrapbook with plain pages and let the kids decorate it. Start by drawing or writing about your favourite foods from different cultures.
3. Plan your first "World Kitchen Wednesday" or whatever day works for you - let your little ones choose a country and help plan the menu. Remember to keep it simple and fun.
4. Visit your local international market or world foods aisle - make it an adventure! Take the kids and let them each pick one new ingredient to try. Pop onto our Facebook group to share what treasures you found.

5 Start your own cultural traditions by borrowing one mealtime custom from another culture - whether it's saying "bon appetit" before meals or using chopsticks for noodles. Practise together!

6 Set up a special space in your kitchen for "international ingredients" - let the kids help organise and label them. They'll feel more connected to trying new foods when they're involved in the process.

7 Create a World Kitchen Passport and start collecting "stamps" for each new cuisine you try. Make it a family challenge to fill it up! Explore by continent, alphabetically or however you want!

8 Pick one simple international dish to make this week - whether it's easy homemade naan bread or simple spring rolls. Remember, it's about the experience, not perfection!

Chapter Twelve

Addressing Common Nutrition Myths

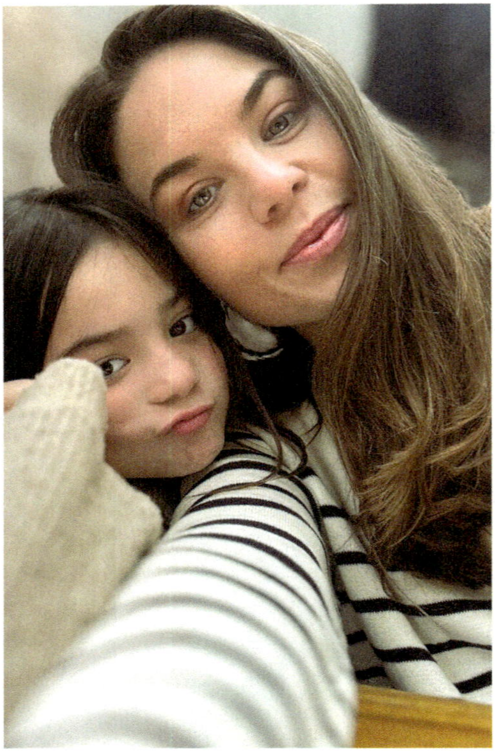

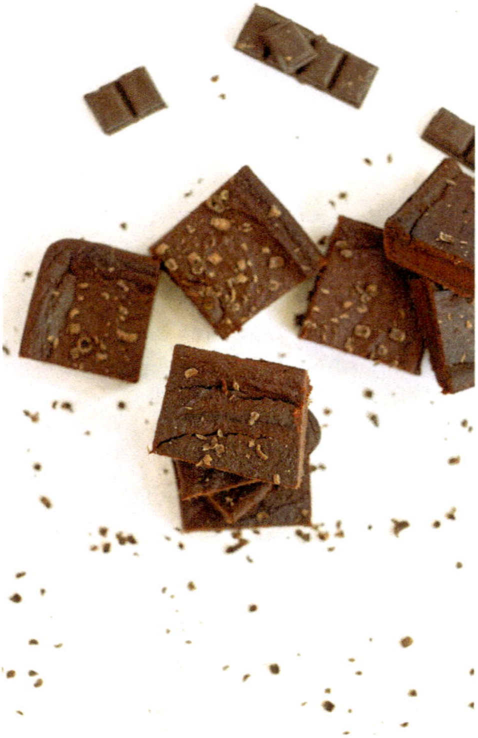

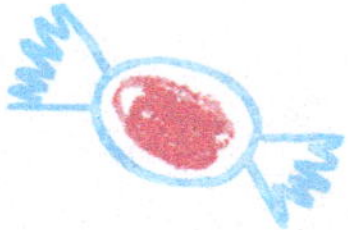

Addressing Common Nutrition Myths

You know those moments when your child catches you sneaking a chocolate biscuit behind the kitchen counter? The other day, Pia found me doing exactly that, and her reaction was priceless: "Mummy, isn't sugar bad for you? That's what you told me!" There I was, caught red-handed by my seven-year-old nutrition police, trying to explain that not all sugar is created equal while simultaneously hiding the evidence of my afternoon treat. It got me thinking about all the nutrition myths floating around and how confusing it must be for parents trying to navigate this minefield of information.

The Sugar Story

Let's talk about sugar, shall we? Because honestly, it's become this huge scary monster in the nutrition world, and I think it's time we brought some sanity back to the conversation. The other day, Pia came home from school absolutely devastated because someone told her that fruit had sugar in it, and now she was worried about eating her beloved strawberries. I had to explain that there was a big difference between the sugar in her strawberries and the sugar in her friend's fruit juices.

Here's the thing about sugar that I wish more people understood: it's not about completely eliminating it from our lives (thank goodness, because I don't think I could survive without my occasional chocolate fix!). It's about understanding the different types and making informed choices. Natural sugars, like those found in fruit and milk, come packaged with all sorts of good stuff, including fibre, vitamins and minerals. When Pia eats an apple, she's not just getting the sugar; she's getting

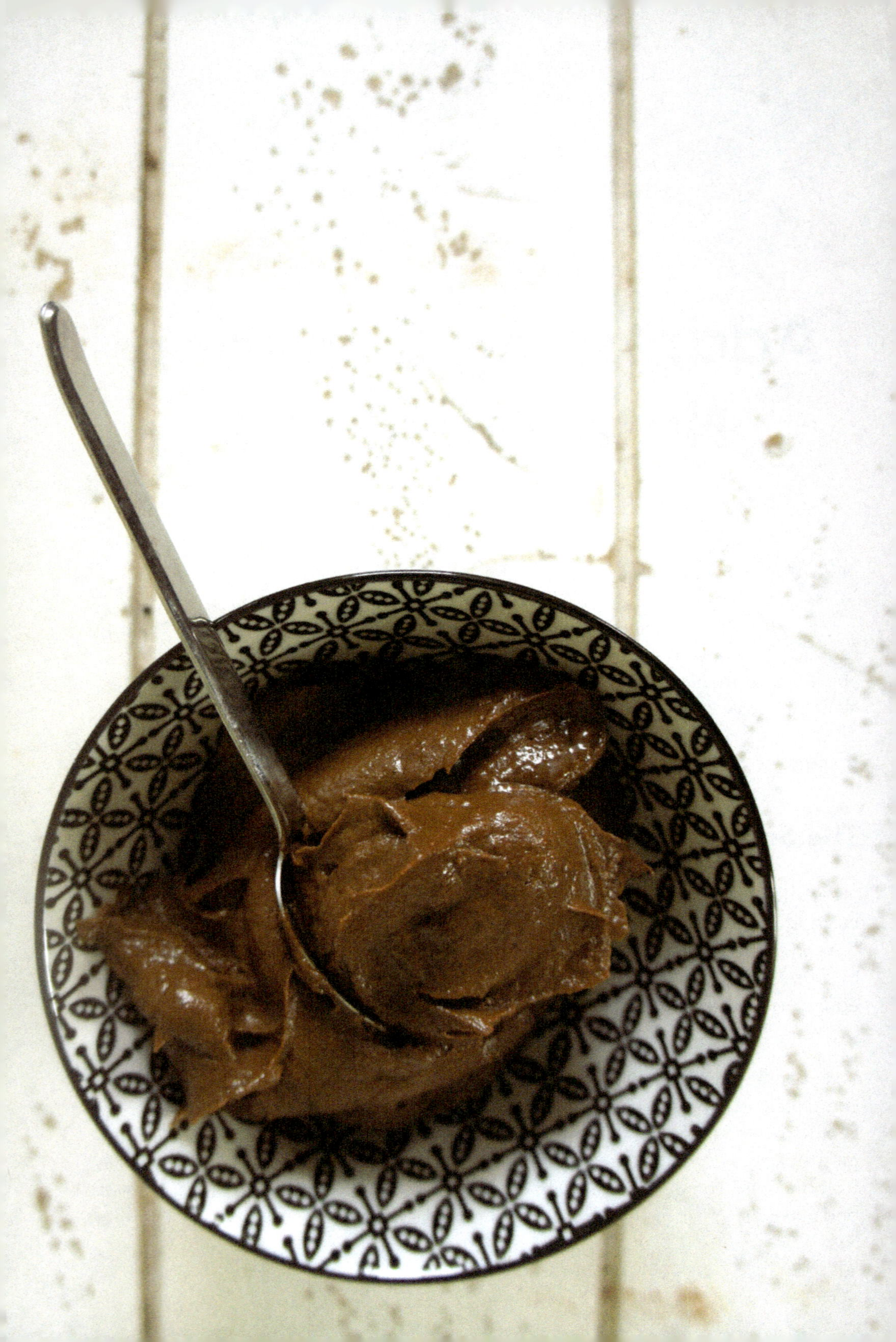

AVOCADO CHOCOLATE MOUSSE

Prep: 10 Mins

Serves 4

2 ripe avocados

1/4 cup unsweetened cocoa powder

1/4 cup honey or maple syrup (adjust to taste)

1/4 cup milk of choice (dairy or plant-based)

1 tsp vanilla extract

A pinch of salt

Optional Toppings

Fresh berries (strawberries, raspberries, or blueberries)

Chocolate chips or shavings

Whipped cream (dairy or coconut)

Sprinkle of colourful sprinkles or mini marshmallows

This avocado chocolate mousse is smooth, chocolaty, and so much fun for kids to make and eat!

Instructions

Prep the Avocados (Kid's Job!): Cut the avocados in half and remove the pits (grown-up step). Let kids scoop out the avocado flesh into a mixing bowl or food processor.

Add Ingredients (Kid's Job!): Help them measure the cocoa powder, honey, milk, vanilla extract, and a pinch of salt. Then, let them add these ingredients to the bowl or food processor with the avocado.

Blend (Grown-Up Step): Blend everything together until it's smooth and creamy. Pause halfway to let kids "taste-test" the mousse. They can add a bit more honey if they want it sweeter or a splash more milk if they want it a bit smoother.

Serve & Decorate (Kid's Job!): Spoon the mousse into small bowls or cups. Then, let the kids add their favourite toppings—berries, chocolate chips, sprinkles, or a dollop of whipped cream. Let them get creative with their designs!

Chill & Enjoy: You can serve it immediately or chill it in the fridge for about 15-20 minutes for an extra-cool treat.

CLEMMIE'S *Tip*

Spoon Tasting: Let kids taste-test along the way with their own spoons and describe the flavour!

Silly Toppings Bar: Set up a little toppings bar where kids can choose and sprinkle on whatever they like.

Make It Fancy: For a fun twist on presentation, serve the mousse in small cups or glass jars, or let kids fill little ice cream cones.

a whole package of nutrients that help her body process that sugar properly.

When I first started studying nutrition, the sugar debate was raging. Everyone was jumping on the "sugar is evil" bandwagon, and honestly, it was exhausting. But here's what I've learned, both as a nutritionist and as a mum: demonising any food or nutrient just creates anxiety and confusion. Instead, I try to help Pia understand that different foods serve different purposes in our bodies.

The other week, we did a little experiment in the kitchen. I showed Pia how many sugar cubes were in her favourite juice compared to a glass of milk. Her eyes nearly popped out of her head! But instead of making her feel guilty about enjoying the occasional juice, we talked about making conscious choices. Now she understands why I'm happy for her to drink milk regularly but saves the juice for special occasions.

The Fat Files Or How I Learned to Love Avocados

Can we talk about fats for a minute? This is another area where there's so much confusion. I still remember the low-fat phase in the 90s—everything was "light" this and "fat-free" that. Here I am, actively trying to get more healthy fats into Pia's diet! The irony isn't lost on me.

Last week, Pia watched me putting avocado in her chocolate mousse (it honestly tastes amazing), and her face was a picture of horror. "Mummy, why are you ruining it?" she wailed. But after tasting it, she couldn't believe that something so creamy and delicious could come from "green mush." It opened up this brilliant conversation about how different types of fats help our bodies in various ways.

I've learned that teaching kids about fats is a bit like teaching them about characters in a story - there are goodies and baddies, but most fall somewhere in between. The healthy fats, like those in olive oil, nuts, and yes, our friend the avocado, are like the superheroes of the nutrition world. They help our brains work better, keep our skin glowing, and even help us absorb essential vitamins. Then there are the not-so-great fats, like trans fats in some processed foods, which are a bit like the villains we try to avoid.

Pia now has this cute way of asking if foods have "superhero fats" in them. The other day, she proudly announced that salmon has "omega-3 superhero powers" - I might have teared up a little at that moment! It's these small wins that make all the nutrition education worth it.

CLEMMIE'S Tip

Avocado Chocolate Mousse

Here's my delicious and creamy Kid-Friendly Avocado Chocolate Mousse recipe that's easy, healthy, and fun for kids to make! It's quick, requires just a few ingredients, and is a perfect treat or dessert.

Check our recipes on our YouTube channel or scan the QR code.

The Organic Dilemma

Oh, the organic debate! I wrestle with this every time I go shopping. I stand in the supermarket, staring at two identical-looking carrots with very different price tags, wondering if the organic one is really worth the extra money. I'll be honest - sometimes, I feel like I need a degree in economics alongside my nutrition qualification to figure this one out!

The other day, Pia asked me why some strawberries cost more than others when they look exactly the same. So we spoke about farming, pesticides, and taking care of our planet. I tried to explain it in a way she'd understand: "Think of it like washing your hands - sometimes you use just water (conventional farming), and sometimes you use soap (organic farming). Both clean your hands, but one might do a more thorough job."

The debate between organic and conventional food can be overwhelming. While organic produce is often considered healthier, it can be more expensive and less accessible. As a busy mum, I've found a practical approach that balances health and budget.

I follow the "Clean 15 and Dirty Dozen" list. This guide highlights the fruits and vegetables with the highest and lowest pesticide residues. For the "Dirty Dozen," I prioritise buying organic to reduce exposure to harmful chemicals. These typically include strawberries because they tend to absorb more pesticides (and because Pia would eat her body weight in them if I let her!), along with spinach and kale. For the "Clean 15," like bananas and avocados, I'm less concerned about organic, as their thicker skin often protects them. By following this approach, I can make informed choices about what I buy without feeling overwhelmed or breaking the bank. It's a simple way to prioritise health and sustainability in our family's diet.

The Supplement Saga

Let me tell you about the time I found Pia trying to convince her little cousin that her gummy vitamin was a magical sweet that would give her superpowers! While I explained that vitamins aren't magical (much to their disappointment), it opened up an interesting discussion about when supplements are helpful and when they're just expensive wee (keeping it real here!).

As a nutritionist and a mother, I have a somewhat conflicted relationship with supplements. On one hand, I know that getting nutrients from whole foods is always the best option. There's something special about how nature packages vitamins and minerals together that we can't replicate in a pill. But on the other hand, I also know that sometimes life (and picky eating phases!) gets in the way of perfect nutrition.

Take vitamin D, for instance. Living in the UK means we're all a bit short on sunshine, especially during those long winter months when the sun seems to forget we exist. So yes, Pia takes a vitamin D supplement during winter, just like most kids should. But do I rely on it as a substitute for healthy eating? Absolutely not.

I remember one mum at school asking me if she could just give her child a multivitamin instead of trying to get them to eat vegetables. Oh, how I wished it was that simple! I had to explain that while supplements can be helpful, they're more like backup singers than the lead vocalists in the nutrition band. They're there to support, not to steal the show!

Seeing as this is a question I get asked a lot, I thought I'd share a list of supplements that are often beneficial for children, along with reasons why each can be helpful. For my recommended suppliers, you can refer to Chapter 14.

CLEMMIE'S Tip

Multivitamin: The benefits they provide is a balanced mix of essential vitamins and minerals that support overall growth, immune health, and energy levels, especially if kids are picky eaters or have dietary restrictions. Sprays work really well.

CLEMMIE'S Tip

Vitamin D: Essential for bone health, immune function, and overall mood support. Since kids don't always get enough sunlight exposure, a supplement can help maintain healthy levels.

CLEMMIE'S Tip

Omega-3 Fatty Acids (DHA/EPA): Important for brain development, cognitive function, and heart health. Omega-3s are typically found in fish, so a supplement is especially helpful if kids don't eat seafood regularly.

CLEMMIE'S Tip

Probiotics: Supports healthy digestion, boosts the immune system, and supports mood. Probiotics help maintain a balanced gut microbiome, which can be beneficial for kids with occasional digestive issues.

CLEMMIE'S Tip

Calcium: Essential for bone and teeth development. Many kids don't get enough calcium from food alone, so a supplement can help meet daily needs.

CLEMMIE'S Tip

Magnesium: Known to support relaxation, sleep, muscle function, and overall mood. Magnesium can be especially helpful for active kids and those who need support with restful sleep.

CLEMMIE'S Tip

Vitamin C: Boosts the immune system, helps the body absorb iron, and supports healthy skin. Vitamin C is an excellent supplement, particularly during cold and flu season.

CLEMMIE'S Tip

Iron (if needed): Important for energy, growth, and oxygen circulation in the blood. Children who are on vegetarian diets or have low energy levels might benefit from additional iron, but always consult a healthcare provider before starting.

If you're feeling unsure about which supplements might be best for your child's unique needs, I offer personalised support to help guide you. You can reach out to me directly through my website for tailored advice and recommendations!

Real Talk About Reading Labels

I'm like a detective in the supermarket, scrutinising labels like I'm trying to crack a code. Pia mostly finds it 'boring' because it admittedly takes twice as long to shop. Still, the other day, she announced very loudly in the yoghurt aisle that we needed to "check for sneaky sugars" - I've never been more proud (or slightly embarrassed)!

Food labels can be incredibly misleading. Companies are very clever with their marketing; sometimes, what looks healthy at first glance isn't quite what it seems. I've developed my "label reading cheat sheet," a mental checklist that helps me quickly decide if something makes the cut.

For example, last week, I was looking at two different granolas. One proudly proclaimed "no refined sugar!" on the front, but when I checked the ingredients, it was packed with honey, maple syrup, and apple juice concentrate. Now, these might sound more natural, but they're still pretty much just sugar to our bodies. The other granola had a shorter ingredient list and less total sugar, even though it didn't make any special claims. Guess which one came home with us?

Making Peace with Food

Let's have a candid moment here. The other day, at a birthday party, I watched as several mums huddled in the corner, whispering about the cake's sugar content and debating whether to let their kids have a slice. Meanwhile, I was helping Pia decide between chocolate or vanilla (she went for both - that's my girl!). Here's the thing: as a nutritionist, I understand the concern about sugar. But as a mum, I also understand the importance of not making food feel forbidden or scary!

MY BLACK BEAN BROWNIES

Prep: 30 Mins

Makes 9

1 can (15 oz) black beans, rinsed and drained

2 large eggs

1/3 cup cocoa powder

1/2 cup honey or maple syrup

1/4 cup melted coconut oil or mild olive oil

1/2 tsp vanilla extract

1/2 tsp baking powder

Optional: chocolate chips or mini M&Ms for topping

a few basil leaves for garnish

Instructions

Preheat the Oven (Grown-Up Step): Preheat the oven to 350°F (180°C). Grease an 8x8-inch baking pan or line it with parchment paper.

Mash the Beans (Kid's Job!): Pour the black beans into a large mixing bowl. Kids can mash them with a fork or potato masher until they're as smooth as possible (or let them leave a few chunks for a fudgy texture).

Add Ingredients (Kid's Job!): Help the kids measure and add the eggs, cocoa powder, honey, melted coconut oil, vanilla extract, and baking powder to the bowl. Then, let them pour everything in and mix it with a spoon.

Blend (Grown-Up Step): For an even smoother brownie batter, use a blender or food processor and blend until smooth.

Pour & Decorate (Kid's Job!): Pour the batter into the prepared pan, then let the kids sprinkle chocolate chips or mini M&Ms on top. Let them create fun patterns or smiley faces with the toppings!

Bake (Grown-Up Step): Bake for 20-25 minutes or until a toothpick comes out mostly clean. Let cool before slicing into squares.

CLEMMIE'S *Tip*

Taste Testing: Before adding the cocoa powder or honey, kids can taste the brownies and guess what they will taste like.

Bean Smooshing: Mashing the beans can be really fun—it's a unique step they won't find in regular brownies!

Topping Creativity: Have a toppings station with chocolate chips, M&Ms, or even a few sprinkles for decorating.

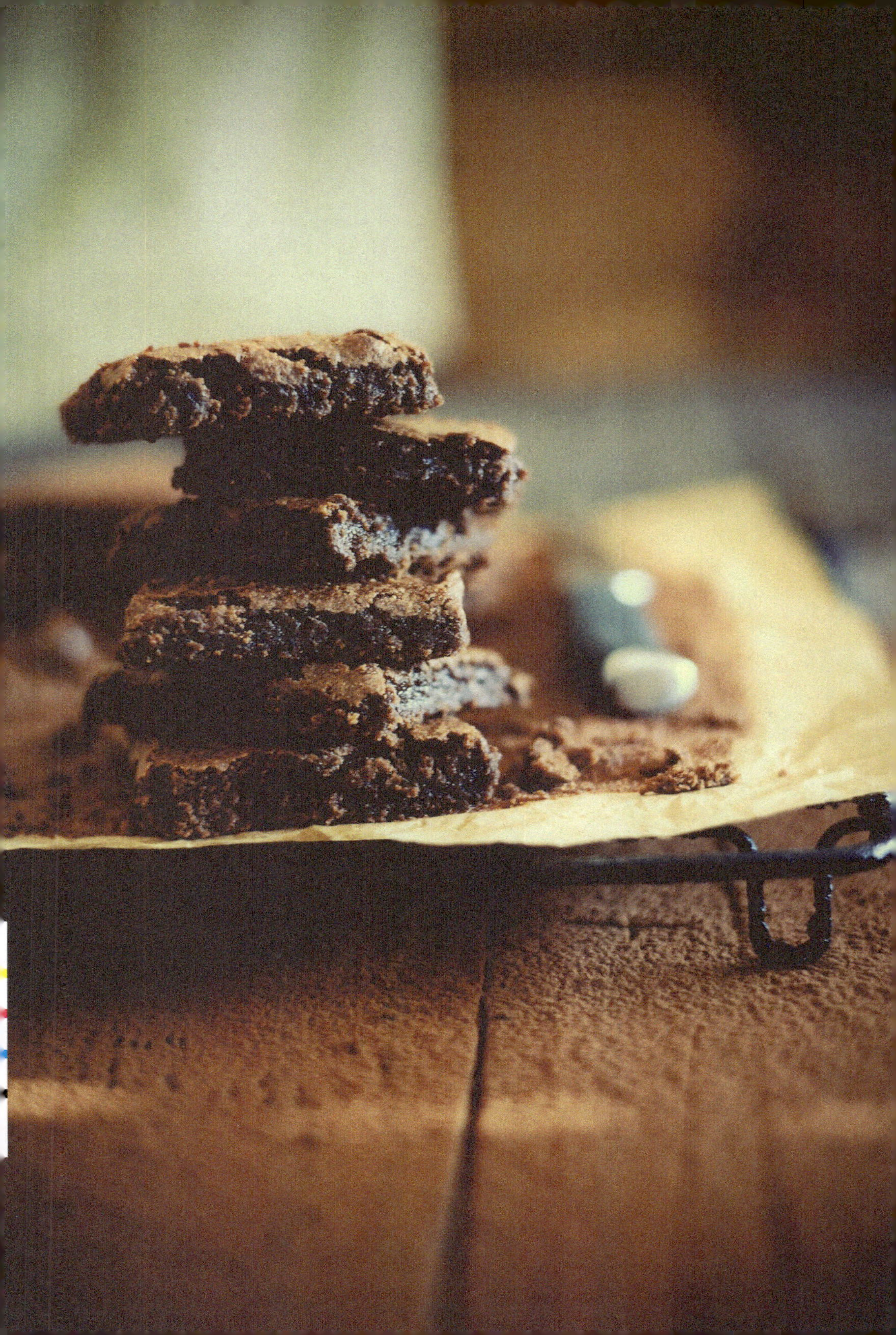

One of the biggest myths about nutrition isn't about specific nutrients - it's the myth that perfect eating exists. It doesn't, and chasing it can do more harm than good, especially when raising children. I want Pia to grow up understanding that food is both fuel and pleasure, that nutrients matter, but so does enjoying a slice of birthday cake with friends.

I decided to get creative in the kitchen the other day and make a "healthy" cake with Pia. We swapped out traditional sugar and flour for healthier alternatives such as Medjool dates and ground almonds. She loved the process and happily ate the remaining raw mixture (a girl after my own heart). However, as soon as we put the batter in the oven, she said, "Right, can we make normal cakes now?" It was a hilarious reminder that sometimes, there's no substitute for the real thing. And that's perfectly okay!

The other week, Pia came home from school upset and confused because someone had told her that bread was "bad." We sat down together, and I explained that her body is like a car - it needs different types of fuel to run properly. Some foods are like everyday fuel that keeps us running smoothly (like our whole grains, fruits, and vegetables), while others are more like premium fuel for special occasions (hello, birthday cake!). Neither is "bad" - they just serve different purposes.

CLEMMIE'S Tip

Black Bean Brownie

Here's a super simple and fun Kid-Friendly Black Bean Brownie recipe that's perfect for kids to join in on. It only uses a few ingredients, and they'll love being able to help blend, mix, and decorate!

Check our recipes on our YouTube channel or scan the QR code.

Finding Your Family's Balance

Through both my professional training and my adventures in motherhood, I've learnt that that balance looks different for every family. In our house, it means having a fruit bowl that is always within reach and keeping some dark chocolate in the cupboard. It means getting excited about trying new vegetables but not freaking out when Pia goes through phases of only wanting pasta (again!).

Last month, we experimented with making healthier versions of our favourite treats. Sometimes, they work brilliantly—like our black bean brownies, which Pia swears are better than regular ones (winning!). And sometimes, they're complete disasters—like when we tried to make "chickpea cookies" that tasted like cooked, sweet hummus. However, these kitchen experiments have taught Pia more about food and nutrition than any lecture ever could.

What to Do Next

1. Spend one week simply noticing (without judgment!) how many different types of foods your family eats. You might be surprised as to which is the most and least recorded!

2. Pick one "processed" food your family loves and read its label together. Don't try to change anything yet; just be curious about what's in it.

3. Choose one new "whole food" to try each week - it could be as simple as a different type of fruit or a new variety of nuts. Ask your little one what they like most about it.

4. Create a "Healthy Fats" shopping list. Start with two or three foods rich in good fats that your family already enjoys, and find a couple for recipes that use them to provide some variety.

5. Plan one "Kitchen Adventure" this week. Try a new recipe or experiment with making a healthier version of a family favourite. Don;t be afraid to fail. Half the fun is trying things together.

6. Check your supplements (if you use them). Are they still needed? If you're unsure, schedule a chat with me, and I can make recommendations.

Chapter Thirteen

Long-Term Impact and Community Building

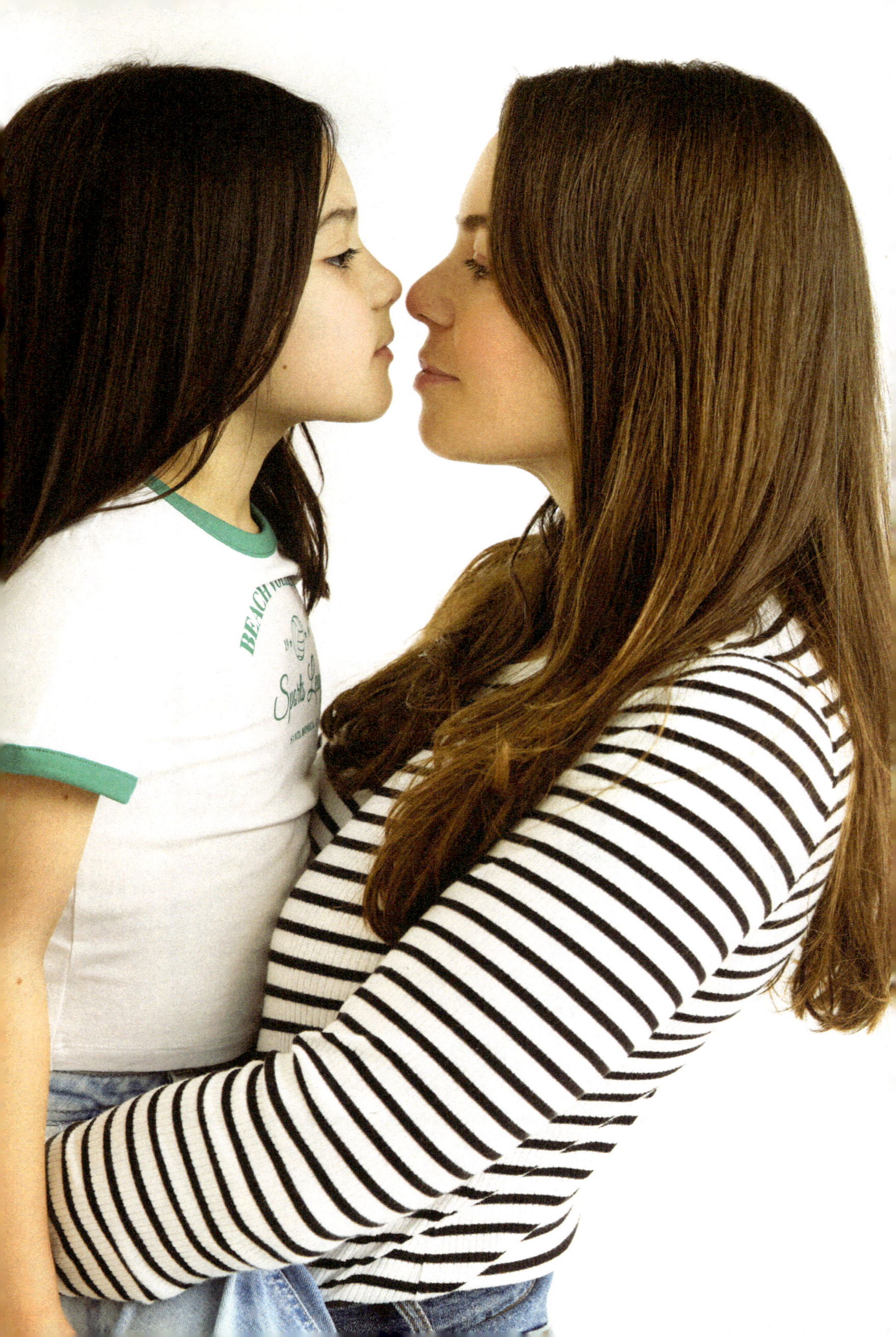
BEACH

Long-Term Impact and Community Building

You know that saying about it taking a village to raise a child? Well, it also takes a village to raise a healthy eater. The other day, I sat in our local park watching Pia play with her friends, chatting with some other mums about the eternal struggle of getting vegetables into reluctant toddlers. I shared my trick about making "rainbow pasta" by blending different vegetables into the sauce, and suddenly, everyone was taking notes on their phones. That's when it hit me - we're all figuring this out together, and there's something really reassuring about that.

Finding Your People

It all started with a desperate message I saw in a huge WhatsApp mum's group I'm a part of: "Anyone else's child suddenly refusing to eat anything green? Help!" Within minutes, my phone was buzzing with responses. Before I knew it, we had inadvertently created (yet another!) a group of mums sharing recipes, wins, and sometimes just sympathetic emojis when dinner ended up on the floor (again).

What began as casual meetups in my kitchen, with kids running around and mums swapping nutrition tips over coffee, has grown into something really special. We now have monthly meetups where everyone brings a healthy dish to share. The rules are simple: it has to be something your kids actually eat (no aspirational recipes allowed!), and you have to be willing to share your secrets when someone's child unexpectedly devours your dish.

Last month, a friend brought these fantastic sweet potato brownies that had all

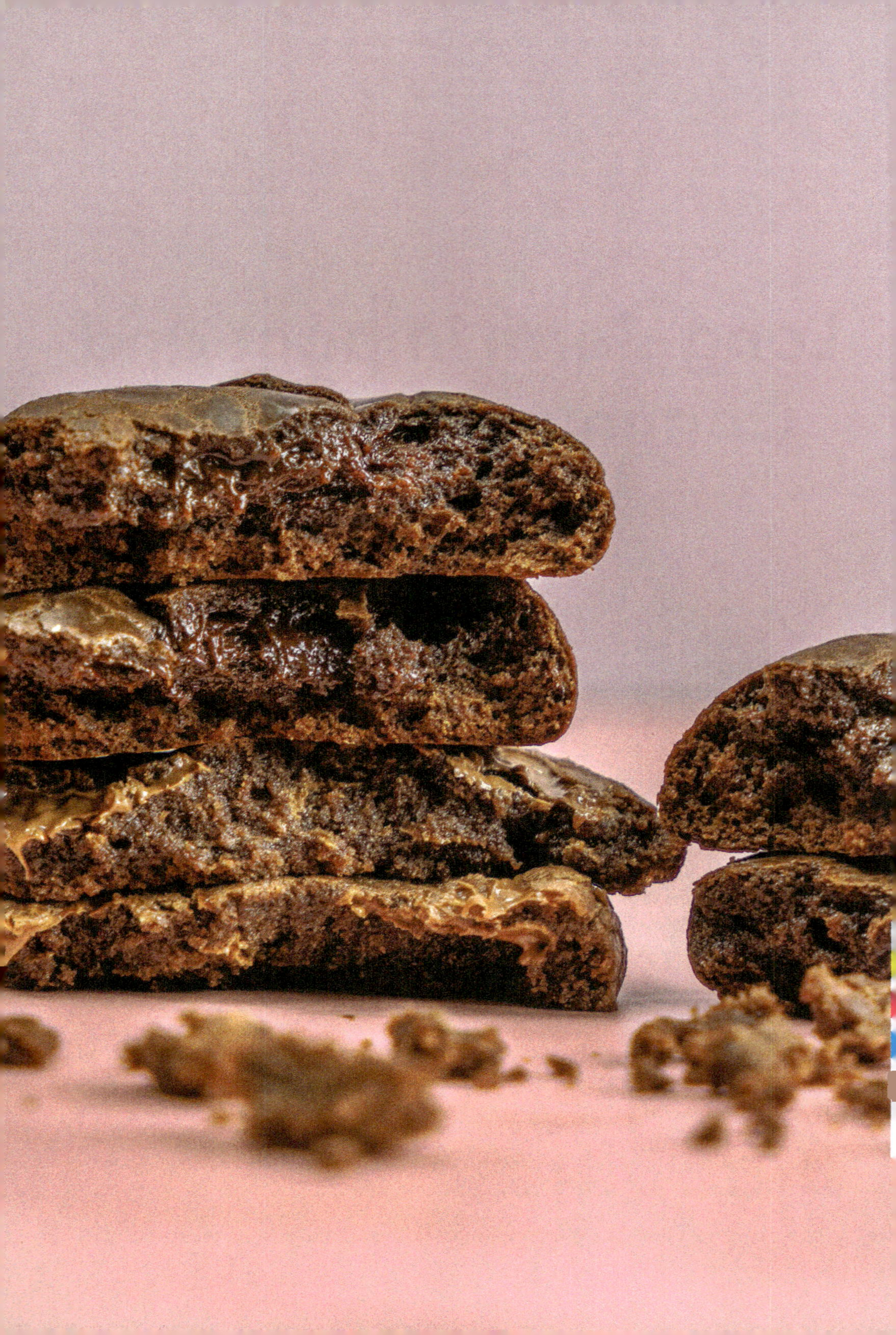

SWEET POTATO BROWNIES

Total: 35 Mins

Makes 9

- 1 medium sweet potato (about 1 cup mashed)
- 1/3 cup cocoa powder
- 1/4 cup honey or maple syrup
- 1/4 cup almond butter (or peanut butter)
- 2 large eggs
- 1 tsp vanilla extract
- 1/2 tsp baking powder
- Pinch of salt
- Optional: 1/4 cup chocolate chips or chopped nuts for topping

Instructions

Preheat the Oven (Grown-Up Step): Preheat the oven to 350°F (175°C). Grease or line an 8x8-inch baking pan with parchment paper.

Cook the Sweet Potato (Kid's Job!): Peel and chop the sweet potato into cubes, then steam or microwave it until tender (about 10 minutes). Let the kids mash it with a fork or potato masher once it's soft.

Mix the Wet Ingredients (Kid's Job!): In a bowl, let the kids mix the mashed sweet potato with the honey or maple syrup, almond butter, eggs, and vanilla extract. Stir until it's all combined.

Add the Dry Ingredients (Kid's Job!): Add the cocoa powder, baking powder, and a pinch of salt to the wet mixture. Let the kids stir everything together until the batter is smooth.

Pour and Decorate (Kid's Job!): Pour the brownie batter into the prepared pan. If you're using chocolate chips or nuts, sprinkle them on top and press them into the batter gently.

Bake (Grown-Up Step): Bake in the preheated oven for about 20-25 minutes or until a toothpick comes out clean (it should still be moist but not gooey). Let cool before slicing.

CLEMMIE'S *Tip*

Sweet Potato Mashing: Let kids really get involved with the mashing! They'll love squashing the soft, sweet potato.

Topping Station: Set up a toppings station with chocolate chips, nuts, or even cinnamon, and let the kids decorate the brownies however they like.

Taste Testing: Kids can taste the honey or maple syrup before mixing it in to guess what flavours are going into the brownies.

our kids fooled. She'd barely finished plating them up before a pack of enthusiastic six-year-olds demolished them. The best part was watching the kids' faces when we told them they'd just eaten vegetables! Though I'm pretty sure, Pia still doesn't believe me about that one.

CLEMMIE'S Tip

Sweet Potato Brownies

These brownies are rich, fudgy, and full of hidden goodness! Plus, they're a fun, interactive way for kids to get involved in the kitchen while making something healthy and tasty. Enjoy!

Check our recipes on our YouTube channel or scan the QR code.

Interactive Element: Community Connection Checklist

Create a checklist of potential local and online communities to explore, including tips on engaging with and contributing positively to each. List events, social media groups, or community boards where you might find your tribe. Consider setting goals for how often you want to connect and engage with these groups. This will help keep your commitment high and your motivation strong.

The Ripple Effect

Here's something I never expected: watching how our family's food choices have started influencing others, primarily through Pia. The other day, she went to a playdate at her friend's house and apparently spent the entire afternoon teaching her friend's mum how to make our "green man smoothie". She even explained why we add leafy greens (which she calls "ninja leaves" because you can't taste them) - I nearly burst with pride when I heard about that!

It's fascinating how children can become the most potent advocates for healthy eating, often without even realising it. Last week at school pickup, another mum told me her daughter now insists on having a "rainbow plate" at dinner because that's what Pia told her about at lunch. This is such a strong reminder that every positive choice we make doesn't just affect our family - it creates ripples extending far beyond our dinner table.

Kitchen Adventures: Labs

Remember when playdates just meant throwing some snacks in a bowl and hoping for the best? Our house has somehow become a "Fun Food Lab" - though I suspect that might have something to do with the time we accidentally made exploding smoothies (note to self: don't blend fizzy water!).

It started quite accidentally, really. One rainy afternoon, I had four restless kids at my house, and in a moment of desperation, I decided to let them help make lunch. Yes, the kitchen ended up looking like a food bomb had gone off, and yes, I found pasta in places it should never have been, but something magical happened. These kids, who usually would turn their noses up at anything resembling a vegetable, were proudly eating the rainbow wraps they'd made themselves.

We were recently making fruit sushi (basically rice-free sushi rolls made with fruit and coconut wraps), and one of the mums brought her son, a particularly picky eater. He started off adamant that he wouldn't touch anything, but watching the other kids having so much fun eventually drew him in. By the end of the session, he was proudly showing off his "dragon roll" (a banana wrapped in mango with berry "scales"). His mum actually cried when he took a bite - those are the moments that make all the mess worthwhile.

When Communities Come Together

We decided to organise a healthy baking workshop at a friend's house, and everything that could go wrong did. The oven decided to have a temperamental moment; someone accidentally used salt instead of sugar (that was actually me - oops!), and one enthusiastic toddler managed to redecorate the walls with beetroot powder. But it became one of our most memorable sessions because everyone pitched in to help fix the chaos. Parents were problem-solving together, kids were giggling at our mistakes, and we all learned that sometimes the biggest disasters make the best stories.

Our next theme is "Around the World in 80 Snacks", where everyone will bring healthy snacks from their cultural backgrounds. Pia wants me to make our favourite Colombian Buñuelos, though she's less enthusiastic about my attempts to recreate them (apparently, Mummy's version is "not quite right", and I agree!).

The Extended Family Challenge

Getting the extended family on board with a plant-based lifestyle can be challenging. I remember the look of horror on my partner's face when I first suggested a partly plant-based Christmas. It was as if I'd suggested cancelling Christmas altogether. But with a little patience and a lot of delicious food, even the most sceptical family members have come around.

You can create so many amazing dishes with vegetables. In fact, my partner, a self-proclaimed veggie sceptic (at the ripe old age of 32!), now happily eats my maple-roasted vegetables as long as they're "soft". Who would have thought?

Celebrating the Small Wins

The other day, I found an old photo from when we first started this journey. It was a picture of Pia's first attempt at making a smoothie bowl - it looked more like swamp soup than the Instagram-worthy creation we'd been trying to copy. Next to it was a photo from last week, in which she'd created this beautiful rainbow bowl topped with fruit and seeds. Looking at those photos side by side reminded me how far we've come.

Sometimes, it's as simple as trying a new vegetable; other times, it's mastering a challenging recipe. Last month, Pia proudly announced that she'd convinced her friend Lucy to try avocado by telling her it was "princess food" because it's green like Tiana's dress from Princess and the Frog. Creative problem-solving at its finest.

The Snowball Effect

What amazes me most about this journey is how one tiny change can create a ripple effect throughout your community. When Pia was at nursery, they had a wonderful tradition of sitting in a circle to try a new fruit or vegetable together. I'll never forget the day Pia came home absolutely buzzing because her whole class had tried dragon fruit! Watching your child become a little nutrition ambassador is truly heartwarming.

These small steps can inspire others to be more adventurous with their food choices. We can create a more food-conscious community by sharing our experiences and encouraging others to try new things.

Creating Lasting Changes

The secret to making these changes stick is making them feel natural rather than forced. In our house, healthy eating has become an ongoing adventure. We are always making healthier versions of our favourite treats. Sometimes, they're wonderful (our black-bean brownies are now famous in our circle), and sometimes, they're... well, let's just say our "cauliflower pizza" phase wasn't quite the success I'd hoped for!

But even the failures have become part of our story. That time, we tried to make "healthy" gummy bears and ended up as rubber bouncy balls. It's now a favourite dinner table story that has everyone in stitches. These moments of laughter and shared experiences are what make the journey memorable and sustainable.

Building Your Legacy -One Meal at a Tim

The other day, I overheard Pia playing with her dolls, setting up a pretend café where she explained the importance of "eating rainbows" and "superhero foods". It was a heartwarming moment that made me realise the profound impact we're having on the next generation. Every meal and conversation shapes their relationship with food and health. We're not just changing our own habits; we're creating a new normal for our children.

Last week, I caught up with my client, whose son used to survive on white pasta and is now actively involved in planning their weekly "colour challenge" meals and cooking alongside her. It's a beautiful example of how small changes can ripple through families. This isn't just a heartwarming story.

What to Do Next

1. Find Your Tribe: Join local or online communities of like-minded parents to share experiences, recipes, and tips. You are of course welcome to come and joi us on our dedicated Facebook page.
2. Host Playdate Cooking Sessions: Turn playdates into fun cooking sessions. Let kids experiment with healthy ingredients and create their own dishes.
3. Embrace Community: Organise community events like cooking workshops or potlucks to share healthy recipes and inspire others, and be somebody that helps to foster the community spirit
4. Lead by Example: Be a role model for your children. Incorporate healthy eating habits into your daily life and share your passion for food.
5. Encourage Exploration: Expose your children to a variety of flavours and textures. Encourage them to try new foods and ask questions about their origin.
6. Turn Cooking into a Family Affair: Involve your family in meal planning and preparation. Make it a fun and interactive experience and live in the moment!
7. Celebrate Small Wins: Acknowledge and celebrate your family's progress, no matter how small. Positive reinforcement can motivate you to keep going.

8. Learn and Grow Together: Continue to educate yourself about nutrition and healthy eating. Share your knowledge with others and learn from their experiences.

Thank you

Thank you so much for taking the time to read this book. Writing it has an amazing process and I truly believe that every family deserves to thrive with the right support and knowledge. If I can help just one family, make one small shift, or inspire one child to embrace healthier habits, then I've done my job.

Every step we take, no matter how small, has the potential to create lasting, positive change. I hope this book has given you some tools, inspiration, and motivation to make those changes. I'd love to see how you're implementing these ideas in your own life! Feel free to share your journey on Instagram or Facebook. I'll always re-share your posts to celebrate your progress and amplify the positive impact. Let's inspire each other!

If you ever feel like you need personalised support or guidance along the way, I'm here to help. Don't hesitate to reach out through my website - together, we can make these changes even more impactful for you and your family.

Thank you again, and I wish you and your loved ones all the best on this exciting journey toward healthier, happier living.

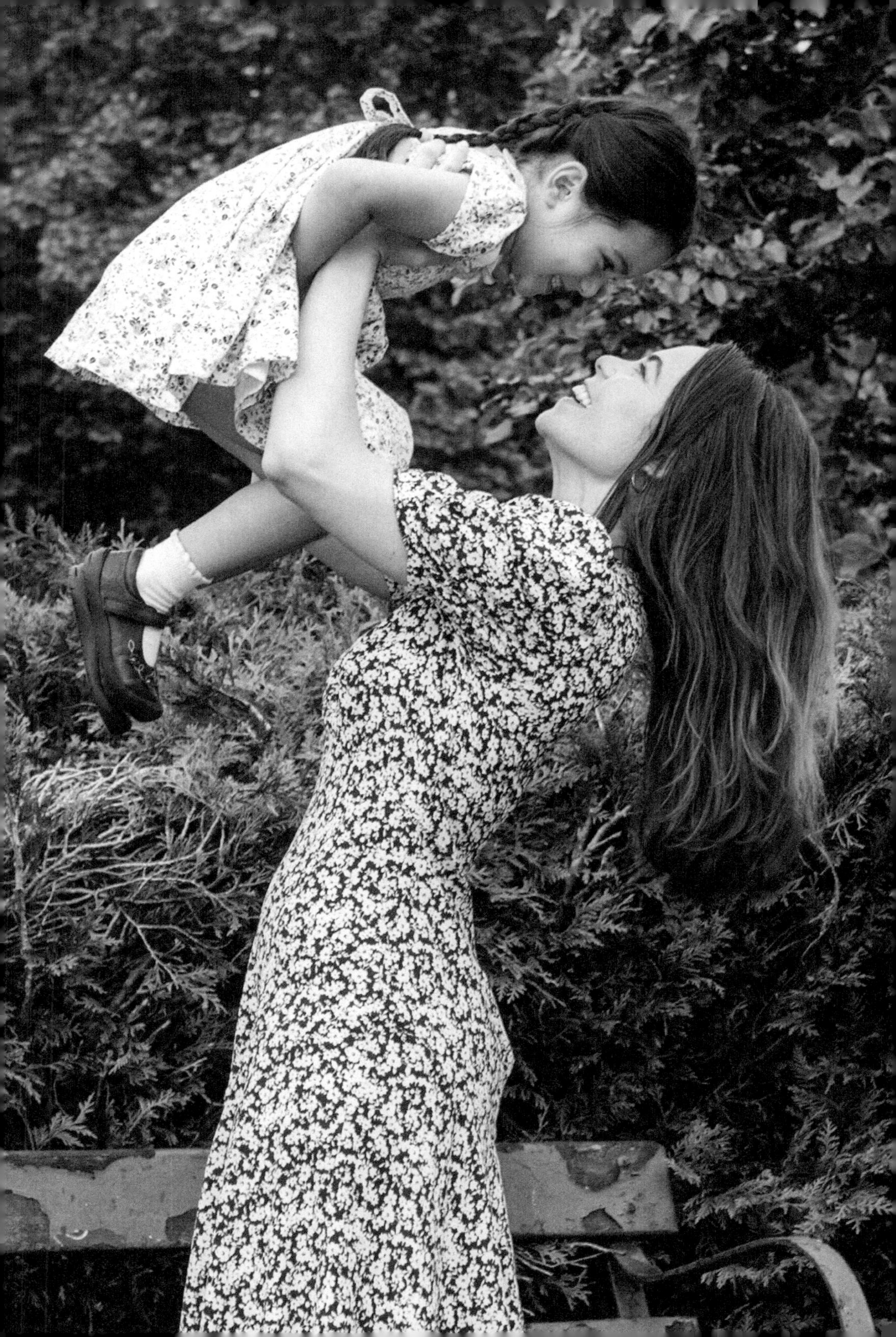

Chapter Fourteen

My Favourite Suppliers

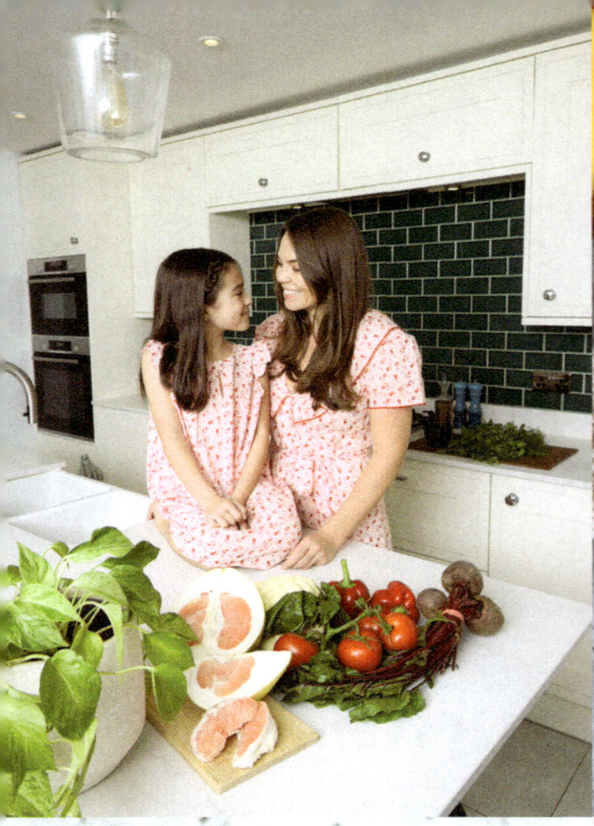
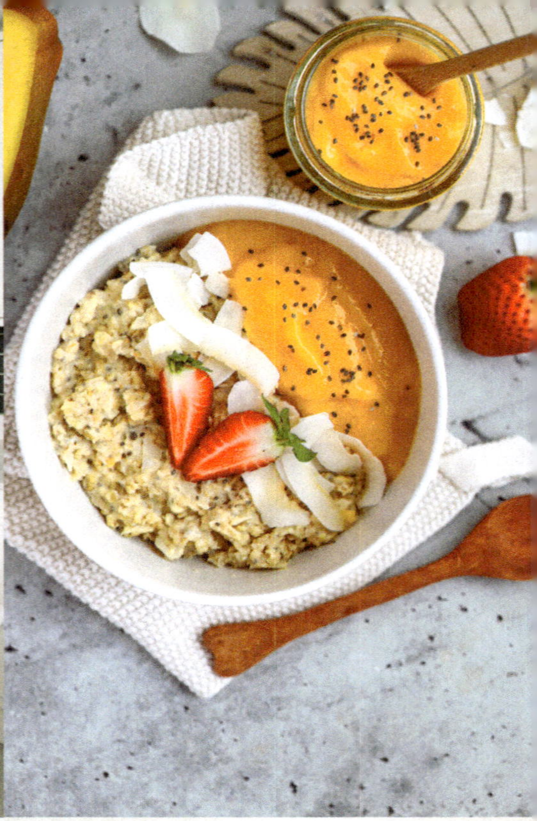
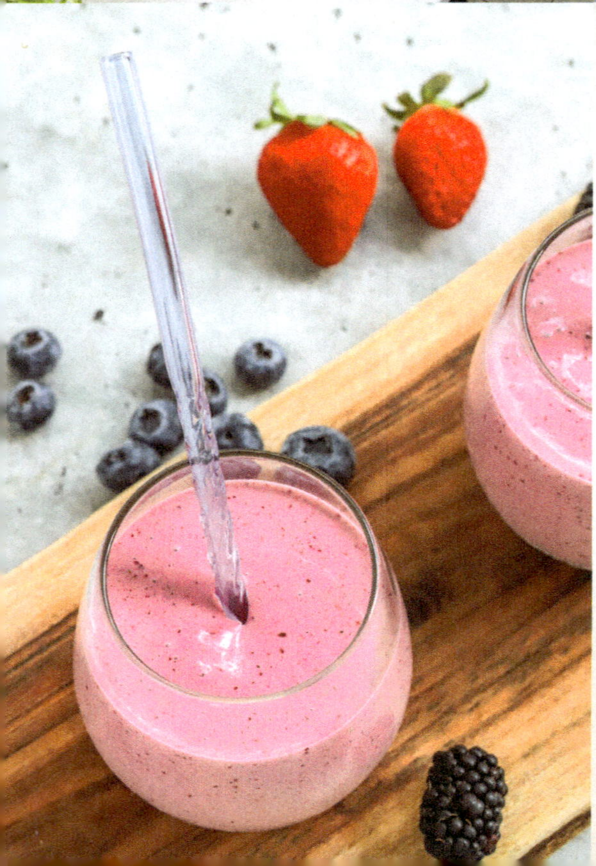
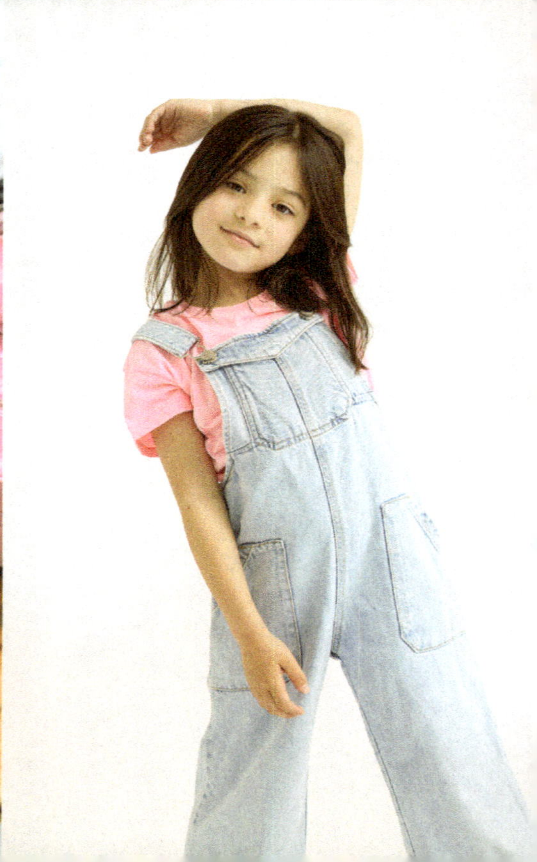

My Favourite Suppliers

Supplements

Symprove Probiotics

Description: Symprove's gentle probiotics support a happy gut for kids. With a mild taste and simple morning routine, it's easy for kids to incorporate, helping them maintain good digestion and energy throughout the day.

Discount: 50% off with discount code.

Website: https://www.symprove.com/

WelleCo Super Elixir for Kids

Description: This nutrient-dense powder is packed with vitamins, minerals, and greens tailored for kids' needs. Simply mix it with water, juice, or smoothies to give kids a daily boost for their immune health and energy.

Website: https://www.welleco.co.uk/

Purition Wholefoods Protein powder

Description: This nutrient-packed powder made from seeds, nuts, and fruits can be added to smoothies, milk, or oats, making it a delicious and healthy treat that kids will love! It's great for a breakfast boost or a snack with protein and fiber.

Discount: 10% off your first order using code **CLEMMIE10.**

Website: https://www.purition.co.uk/

Balance Coffee - Mushroom Tinctures

Description: Balance Coffee's mushroom drops are a quick, easy way to add nutrients to smoothies or juice. Each blend supports focus, immunity, or calm—perfect for busy or energetic little ones needing a natural boost.

Discount: Use code **CLEMMIE20** for a 20% off your first order

Website: https://balancecoffee.co.uk/collections/mushroom-tincture-drops

The Natural Dispensary - Kid-Friendly Supplements

Description: The Natural Dispensary offers a huge range of children's supplements including multivitamins and immune support. These options are perfect for little ones needing extra nutritional support to complement their daily diet.

Discount: Use code **CPHROSE10** for a 10% discount.

Website: https://naturaldispensary.co.uk/

Food

Pip&Nut - Almond Butter

Description: This smooth almond butter is just almonds and a pinch of salt—perfect for adding protein and healthy fats to snacks and meals. Try it spread on toast, stirred into oatmeal, or paired with fruit slices.

Discount: Use code **CLEMENTINEROSENUTRITION** for a 20% off selected collections (excluding sales items)

Website: https://www.pipandnut.com/

Pip Organic

Description: Pip Organic's fruity drinks and snacks are made from real organic fruits, giving kids a naturally sweet treat with no added sugars. Perfect for lunchboxes, they offer a fun way to enjoy fruit on the go.

Website: https://piporganic.com/

Little Dish

Description: Little Dish creates ready-made meals for toddlers and young kids, using real ingredients like vegetables, whole grains, and proteins with no added sugar or artificial ingredients. Each meal is carefully portioned and ready in minutes, perfect for busy families.

Website: https://www.littledish.co.uk/

Ella's Kitchen

Description: Ella's Kitchen offers a wide variety of organic pouches, snacks, and meals for babies and toddlers, using fun flavors and bright packaging to encourage adventurous eating from a young age. Their food is organic, natural, and free from additives.

Website: https://www.ellaskitchen.co.uk/

Piccolo Foods

Description: Piccolo provides organic, nutrient-dense snacks and meal ingredients made with sustainably sourced ingredients. Their products are healthy and convenient for quick meals or snacks, supporting balanced nutrition while prioritizing eco-friendly packaging The pouches also double up as great smoothie boosters!

Website: https://www.mylittlepiccolo.com/

Organix Finger Foods

Description: Organix snacks are designed with little ones in mind, offering organic, easy-to-hold options like veggie sticks, rice cakes, and fruit bars. Perfect for school snacks and lunch boxes - made without artificial additives.

Discount Code: **THANKYOU10**

Website: https://www.organix.com/

Goodies by Organix

Description: Organix's Goodies line offers healthy snacks for kids, from oat bars and fruit snacks to mini rice cakes and savory crackers. All products are organic and made with whole ingredients, perfect for on-the-go munching or lunchbox additions.

Website: https://www.organix.com/

Bear Snacks

Description: Bear Snacks are made from 100% natural fruits, gently baked with no added sugar. Their snack range includes fruit rolls, fruit shapes, and paw prints, making them a fun and wholesome treat for kids of all ages.

Website: https://www.bearsnacks.co.uk/

Cooking tools, Food storage and Lunchboxes

IKEA - Kids Cooking Essentials

Description: IKEA offers great tools for little chefs, including mini aprons and sturdy kitchen steps that allow kids to join in on the cooking fun. These make meal prep interactive and safe, so kids can enjoy hands-on experiences in the kitchen. They also do a great range of glass tupperware.

Website: https://www.ikea.com/gb/en/cat/children-bc003/

Munchkin Bento Boxes

Description: These colorful bento boxes are perfect for keeping kids' snacks and lunches organised. With separate sections, they make it easy to pack a balanced, fun meal that keeps each food fresh and contained.

Website: https://www.munchkin.co.uk/products/lunch-bento-box-with-stainless-steel-utensils?Color=Yellow

Ion Water Bottles

Description: Bright and easy-to-grip, Ion water bottles make hydration fun and convenient for kids. Leak-proof and available in fun colors, they're perfect for taking to school, sports, or playdates.

Website: https://www.ion8.co.uk/collections/water-bottles

PlanetBox Eco-Friendly Lunchboxes

Description: PlanetBox lunchboxes are made from stainless steel and designed to last for years. Each box features compartments that help parents create balanced, visually appealing meals. Their eco-friendly materials reduce waste, and the customizable magnet designs make them especially fun for kids.

Website: https://www.planetbox.com/

Ecozoi Bamboo Cutlery and Plates

Description: Ecozoi offers a range of sustainable, BPA-free bamboo plates, bowls, and utensils perfect for kids. Their products are fully biodegradable and come in cute designs that add a playful touch to mealtime, encouraging kids to eat healthy, all while being eco-friendly.

Website: https://ecozoi.com/

Stasher Reusable Silicone Bags

Description: Stasher bags are made from 100% pure platinum silicone and are a perfect eco-friendly replacement for single-use plastic bags. They're great for packing snacks, sandwiches, and other foods in a colorful, reusable, and dishwasher-safe bag that keeps food fresh.

Website:https://www.stasherbag.com/

WeeSprout Stainless Steel Bento Box

Description: WeeSprout's stainless steel bento boxes are durable, eco-friendly, and perfectly sized for kids. With separate compartments, these boxes help keep meals organised and encourage balanced eating. Their lightweight design makes them ideal for school lunches and snacks.

Website: https://www.weesprout.com/

Keep Leaf Organic Cotton Lunch Bags

Description: Keep Leaf's lunch bags are made from organic cotton and are perfect for packing meals in an eco-friendly, reusable way. Their designs are colorful and child-friendly, making them an attractive alternative to disposable packaging.

Website: https://keepleaf.com/

OXO Tot - Kitchen Tools for Kids

Description: OXO Tot's range of kitchen tools is designed for small hands, including safe knives, measuring cups, and mixing bowls. These tools let kids join in cooking activities safely, teaching them new skills while having fun.

Website: https://www.oxo.com/shop/baby-toddler.html?

MontiiCo Lunch Bags

Description: MontiiCo's fun, insulated lunch bags keep food fresh and come in colourful designs that kids love. The roomy interior makes it easy to pack balanced meals, and it's super easy to clean, too.

Website: https://montii.co/collections/lunch-bags

Yumbox - Leakproof Lunchboxes

Description: Yumbox lunchboxes feature divided sections and a leakproof design, making it fun and easy to pack a variety of foods for kids. The boxes are durable and come in bright colours that add a splash of fun to lunchtime.

Website: https://www.scandibugs.co.uk/collections/yumbox

About The Author

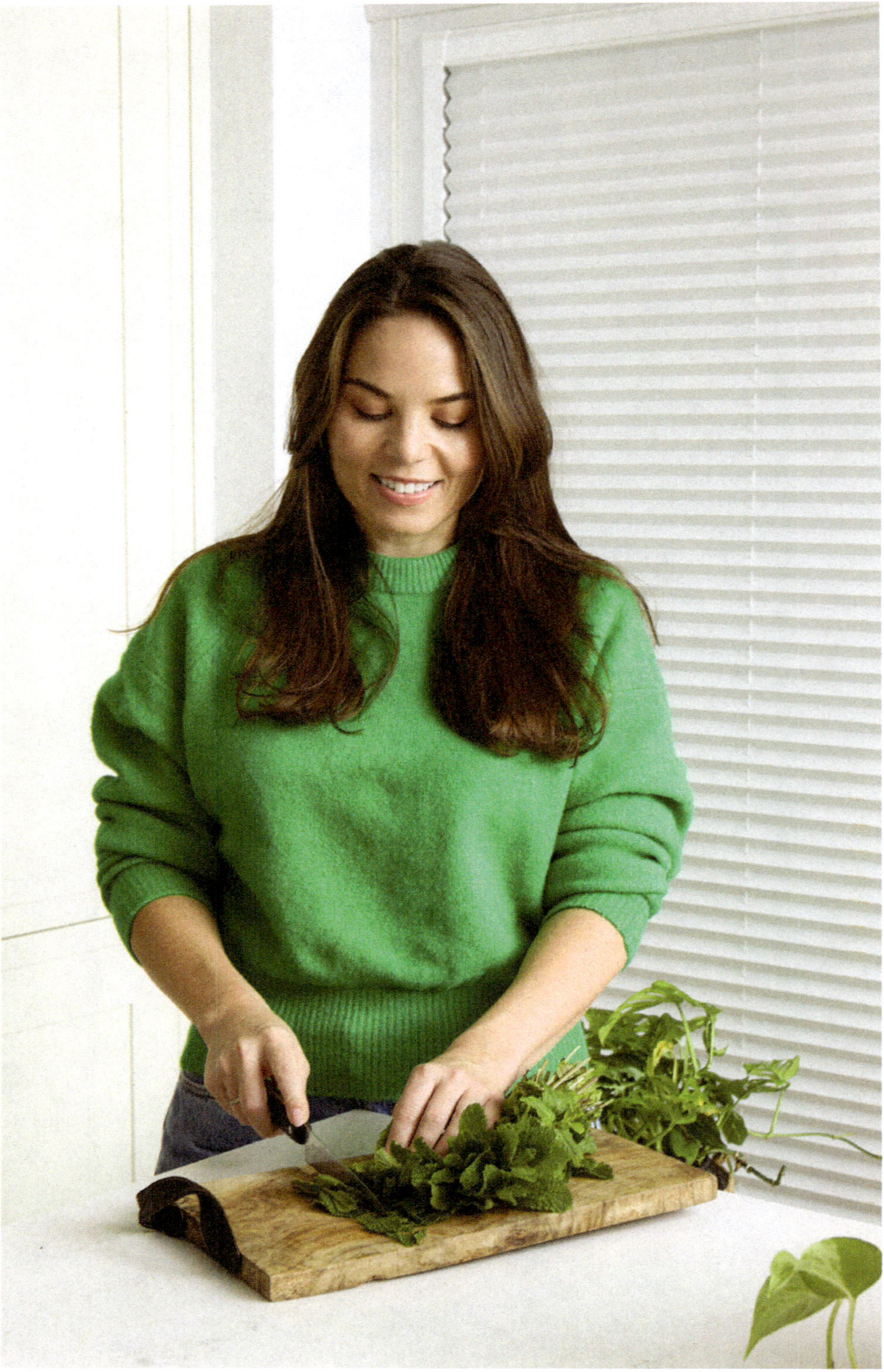

About the Author

Hello! I'm Clementine Pellew-Harvey, but you can call me Clemmie. I'm a qualified Nutritional Therapist based in London, and my passion lies in helping families create a positive relationship with food. I received my training at the College of Naturopathic Medicine in Kings Cross and am proud to be a member of the British Association for Nutrition and Lifestyle Medicine (BANT).

As a mother to my 7-year-old daughter, Pia, I have firsthand experience with the challenges of raising a fussy eater. Navigating mealtime with a picky child can be tough, but I believe a healthy relationship with food starts at home. It's our responsibility to model positive behaviours, and I've learned that the key to success is making food enjoyable and accessible. This personal journey inspired me to write this book, which is my way of sharing what I've learned and offering support to parents facing similar challenges.

I firmly believe that our relationship with food shapes our overall well-being. It's crucial to address disordered eating habits, which often stem from societal pressures and unrealistic expectations. By creating a nurturing environment and enjoyable mealtime experiences, we can help our children develop a healthier outlook on food. My approach goes beyond just the ingredients on the plate; it's about developing connections and joy around meals.

Through my online 1:1 nutrition consultations, I provide personalised guidance tailored to each individual's needs and preferences. I've worked with a diverse range of clients, from high-profile individuals to everyday families seeking to improve their health. My goal is to empower everyone to address the root causes of their eating concerns while developing sustainable habits that support their goals and long-term wellness.

In addition to my private practice, I'm honoured to be part of The Kyros Project, where we utilise advanced biomedical blood testing to help clients gain valuable insights into their health. I also lead nutrition clinics in prestigious locations, including Harrods, Google DeepMind, and clinics in Saudi Arabia. Each of these experiences has enriched my understanding of nutrition and inspired me to continue learning and sharing my knowledge.

This book is a heartfelt resource for parents, reminding you that you're not alone in this journey. Together, we can tackle disordered eating by nurturing our children's love for food and teaching them to listen to their bodies. I believe that creating a supportive and enjoyable mealtime experience can lay the foundation for a lifetime of healthy habits.

To make this an ongoing conversation where we can all help each other, I have set up a dedicated Private Facebook Group for readers of this book, "How To Talk To Kids About Nutrition Group". My hope is that parents will share tips, ideas, stories, and ask whatever is on their mind. In return we share regular features, news and ideas as well as sharing advice, new recipes, supplier discounts and much more. Come and check us out and join in the conversation!

Click to Join the dedicated Facebook group or scan the QR code.

Thank you for joining me on this journey! I'm excited to share my experiences and insights with you, and I hope to inspire families to embrace a wholesome, nourishing approach to eating.

Clemmie

Clemmie Pellew-Harvey
London, November 2024

Leave a Review

"All children should have the basic nutrition they need to learn and grow and to pursue their dreams, because, in the end, nothing is more important than the health and well-being of our children." – Michelle Obama.

I hope that you found the book fun, easy to read and useful. I suspect that there are many Mums out there, who were like you used to be. Less experienced, needing answers, but not sure who or what to trust.

Most people do, in fact, judge a book by its cover (and its reviews). So here's my request to you as an amazing Mum who I know is committed to helping others succeed.

Please help that other Mum by leaving this book a review.

It's remarkably hassle-free, it doesn't cost you anything, it will take about 60 seconds and your review really could help.

If you are on audible - hit the three dots in the top right of your device, click rate & review, then leave a few sentences about the book with a star rating.

If you are reading on kindle, iPad or other tablet - scroll to the bottom of the book, then swipe up and it will prompt a review for you.

If you are reading the Paperback or Hardback version then go to Amazon and leave a review right on the book's page. Use the link or scan the QR Code:

https://geni.us/review-TTK

Thank you for doing that. It makes more of a difference to the next leader who may be considering whether to get this book than you realize.

Clemmie

Clemmie Pellew-Harvey

London, May 2024

Resources

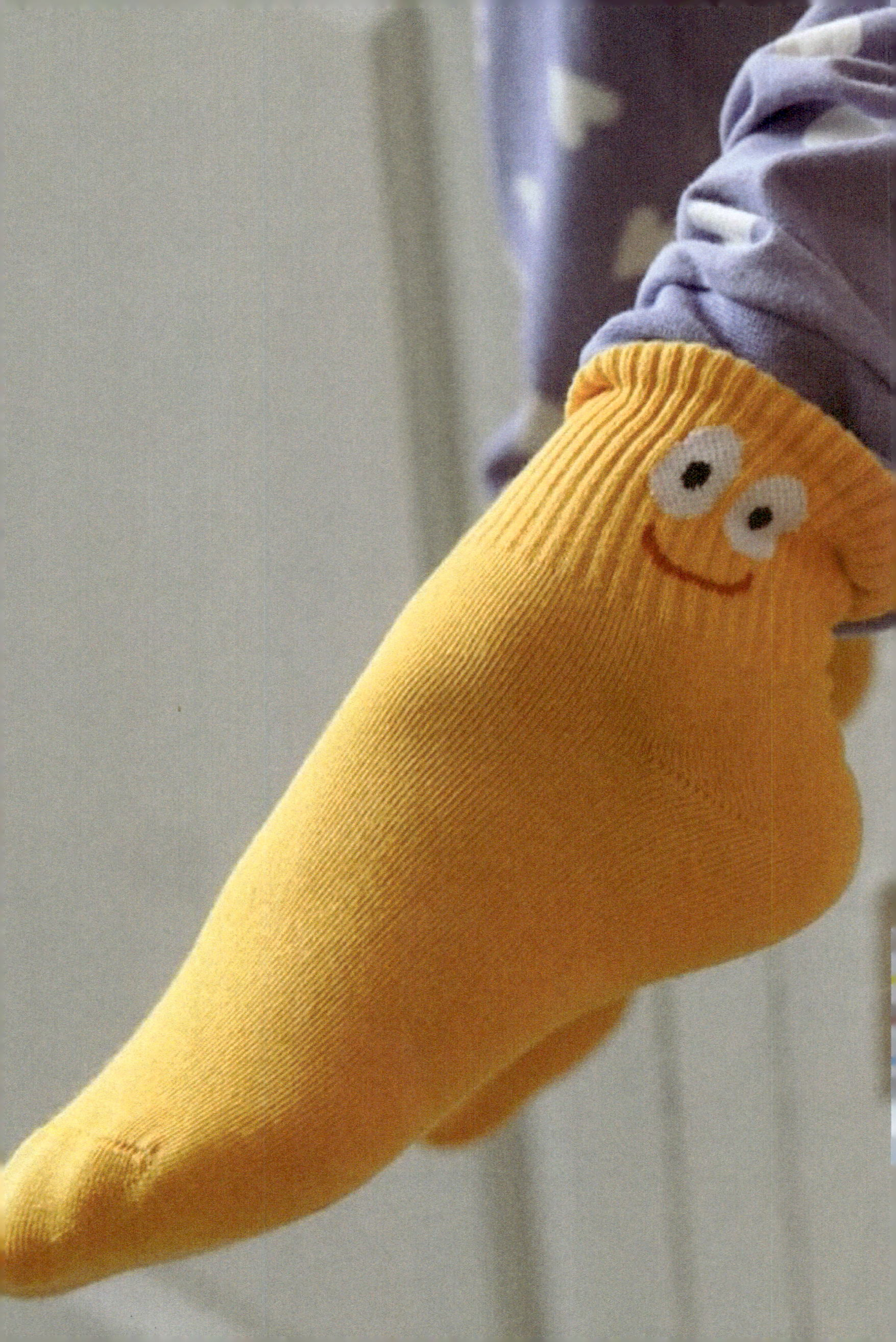

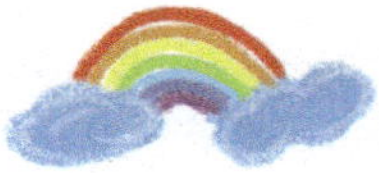

Resources

Mayo Clinic. “What Nutrients Does Your Child Need Now?,” n.d. https://www.mayoclinic.org/healthy-lifestyle/childrens-health/in-depth/nutrition-for-kids/art-20049335.

The Nutrition Source. “Kid's Healthy Eating Plate,” May 9, 2024. https://nutritionsource.hsph.harvard.edu/kids-healthy-eating-plate/.

Johns Hopkins Medicine. “Finding the Hidden Sugar in the Foods You Eat,” June 20, 2024. https://www.hopkinsmedicine.org/health/wellness-and-prevention/finding-the-hidden-sugar-in-the-foods-you-eat.

Taylor, Caroline M., and Pauline M. Emmett. “Picky Eating in Children: Causes and Consequences.” Proceedings of the Nutrition Society 78, no. 02 (November 5, 2018): 161–69. https://doi.org/10.1017/s0029665118002586.

Kids, Pbs. “9 Tips to Help Kids Try New Foods | Parenting Tips & Advice.” PBS KIDS for Parents, April 10, 2024. https://www.pbs.org/parents/thrive/9-tips-to-help-kids-try-new-foods.

ACEQUA, “Creating positive mealtimes”, n.d. https://www.acecqa.gov.au/latest-news/blog/creating-positive-mealtimes

"Raising Healthy Eaters From a Young Age," n.d. https://www.texashealth.org/areyouawellbeing/Family-Health/Raising-Healthy-Eaters-from-a-Young-Age.

Rabinovitch, Lara. "The Best Kids Cooking Tools (That You'll Love Too)." Wirecutter: Reviews for the Real World, October 24, 2024. https://www.nytimes.com/wirecutter/reviews/best-tools-for-cooking-with-kids/.

My Kids Lick The Bowl. "Kid-Friendly-Recipes - My Kids Lick the Bowl," May 31, 2023. https://mykidslickthebowl.com/kid-friendly-recipes/.

Whitefors, Amy, "The Benefits of Cooking with Kids", March 24, 2021 https://www.healthylittlefoodies.com/the-benefits-of-cooking-with-kids/

"Kids Cooking Activities-Ideas, Recipes and Activities to Teach Kids Cooking.," n.d. https://www.kids-cooking-activities.com/.

"Food Allergies | Healthy Schools | CDC," n.d. https://www.cdc.gov/healthyschools/foodallergies/index.htm.

Kids With Food Allergies. "How to Cook for Food Allergies," January 18, 2023. https://kidswithfoodallergies.org/recipes-diet/recipe-substitutions/.

Bernsteinaller. "How to Communicate Allergy Concerns With Teachers and School Administrators - Research Center." Research Center, November 3, 2023. https://www.bernsteinallergyresearch.com/research-center/blog/2023/11/03/how-to-communicate-allergy-concerns-with-teachers-and-school-administrators/.Section 504

Kids With Food Allergies. "Section 504 Plans for Students With Food Allergies | kidswithfoodallergies.org," September 16, 2024. https://kidswithfoodallergies.org/living-with-food-allergies/planning-for-school/section-504-plans-for-students-with-food-allergy/

Pantazi, Alexandru Cosmin, Adriana Luminita Balasa, Cristina Maria Mihai, Tatiana Chisnoiu, Vasile Valeriu Lupu, Mustafa Ali Kassim Kassim, Larisia Mihai, et al. "Development of Gut Microbiota in the First 1000 Days After Birth and Potential Interventions." Nutrients 15, no. 16 (August 20, 2023): 3647. https://doi.org/10.3390/nu15163647.

Oldenburg, Catherine E, Ali Sié, Boubacar Coulibaly, Lucienne Ouermi, Clarisse Dah, Charlemagne Tapsoba, Till Bärnighausen, et al. "Effect of Commonly Used Pediatric Antibiotics on Gut Microbial Diversity in Preschool Children in Burkina Faso: A Randomized Clinical Trial." Open Forum Infectious Diseases 5, no. 11 (November 1, 2018). https://doi.org/10.1093/ofid/ofy289.

Philadelphia, Children's Hospital Of. "Food as Medicine: Probiotic Foods." Children's Hospital of Philadelphia, n.d. https://www.chop.edu/health-resources/food-medicine-probiotic-foods.

National Library of Medicine, "The Molecular Gut-Brain Axis in Early Brain Development:, December 6, 2022, https://www.ncbi.nlm.nih.gov/pmc/articles/PMC9739658/

Blanton, Kayla. "8 Scientific Benefits of Meal Prepping." EverydayHealth.com, October 15, 2024. https://www.everydayhealth.com/diet-nutrition/scientific-benefits-of-meal-prepping/.

Bratskeir, Kate, and James Brains. "The 8 Best Meal Prep Tools to Save You Time and Effort in the Kitchen." Business Insider, January 24, 2024. https://www.businessinsider.com/guides/kitchen/meal-prep-tools.

"Grab-and-go Breakfasts: Chia Pudding and Peanut Butter Yogurt Dip," September 27, 2024. https://www.today.com/health/diet-fitness/healthy-breakfast-ideas-for-kids-rcna98797.

Jawad, Yumna. "40+ Kids Lunch Box Ideas." Feel Good Foodie, July 29, 2023. https://feelgoodfoodie.net/back-school-lunchbox-ideas/.Nutritional Literacy: Teaching Healthy Eating Through Stories https://www.fairygreenwood.com/post/nutritional-literacy-teaching-healthy-eating-through-stories

Charland, Dennis. "10 Best Health & Nutrition Education Apps for Kids." Connecting Communities to the Land, March 4, 2015. https://seewhatgrows.org/10-best-health-nutrition-apps-kids/.Teaching Kids about Culture through Global Cuisine + Recipes http://www.homelifeabroad.com/food-health/recipes/teaching-kids-culture-cuisine/

The Nutrition Source. "Kid's Healthy Eating Plate," May 9, 2024. https://nutritionsource.hsph.harvard.edu/kids-healthy-eating-plate/.

Np, SueMarie Mendez. "Family Wellness: Setting Goals for a Healthy Family." Peak Vista Community Health Centers (blog), n.d. https://www.peakvista.org/blog/family-wellness-setting-goals-for-a-healthy-family.

Ellingwood, Jana. "10 Healthy Family Communication Skills & How to Implement Them." Anchor Light Therapy Collective, June 26, 2024. https://anchorlighttherapy.com/family-communication/.

Wei, Julie. "Meal Planning: A Shared Responsibility." Dr. Julie Wei, February 19, 2019. https://www.drjuliewei.com/blogs/news/meal-planning-a-shared-responsibility.

Momwithfive. "Tips How to Celebrate Health and Wellnes Milestones (2023)." Mom With Five, September 26, 2023. https://www.momwithfive.com/en/2023/09/25/family-celebration-healt-wellness-milestones/.

Teaching kids the art of mindful eating - MSU Extension https://www.canr.msu.edu/news/teaching_kids_the_art_of_mindful_eating

Dawn Earnesty, Michigan State University Extension and Alea Carlson, Central Michigan University Dietetics student. "Teaching Kids the Art of Mindful Eating." MSU Extension, April 20, 2016. https://www.canr.msu.edu/news/teaching_kids_the_art_of_mindful_eating.

"Healthy Eating (for Parents)," n.d. https://kidshealth.org/en/parents/habits.html.

Anne Arundel County Public Schools' Wellness Council. "Why Healthy Rewards?" Anne Arundel County Public Schools' Wellness Policy, 2021. https://aacpsschools.org/nutrition/wp-content/uploads/2024/02/healthy_rewards_students.2023.pdf.

"20 Money-Saving Grocery Shopping Tips," n.d. https://www.eatright.org/food/planning/food-security-and-sustainability/20-money-saving-grocery-shopping-tips.

———. "10 Benefits of Eating Seasonally." Farm Hippie Farmers Market, April 3, 2023. https://farmhippiefarmersmarket.com/10-benefits-of-eating-seasonally/.11 superfoods to boost any kid's diet | BabyCenter https://www.babycenter.com/toddler/feeding/7-superfoods-to-boost-any-kids-diet_10392752

Jenni. “Around the Globe in 80 Meals – Kid Friendly Recipes From Around the World.” The Gingered Whisk, June 26, 2024. https://thegingeredwhisk.com/around-world-80-meals/.

“USDA MyPlate Nutrition Information for Kids,” n.d. https://www.myplate.gov/life-stages/kids.

Doerr, Elizabeth. “The Power of Food in Storytelling — Doerr&Co.” Doerr&Co., August 26, 2021. https://www.doerrandco.com/stories/the-power-of-food-amp-storytelling.

Admin. “Understanding Natural Versus Added Sugars - Center for Healthy Eating and Activity Research.” Center for Healthy Eating and Activity Research (blog), February 26, 2021. https://chear.ucsd.edu/blog/understanding-natural-versus-added-sugars.

PharmD, Jennifer Moll. “Saturated Vs. Unsaturated Fats.” Verywell Health, June 25, 2024. https://www.verywellhealth.com/difference-between-saturated-fats-and-unsaturated-fats-697517.

Rodale Institute. “Organic Vs Conventional - Rodale Institute,” December 3, 2018. https://rodaleinstitute.org/why-organic/organic-basics/organic-vs-conventional/.

Haimi, Motti, and Aaron Lerner. “Nutritional Deficiencies in the Pediatric Age Group in a Multicultural Developed Country, Israel.” World Journal of Clinical Cases 2, no. 5 (January 1, 2014): 120. https://doi.org/10.12998/wjcc.v2.i5.120.

American Heart Asoicaiton. “Healthy for Life”, n.d. https://www.heart.org/en/healthy-living/company-collaboration/healthy-for-life

NY Enrichment Group. “Nutrition Education for Parents | NY Enrichment Group,” n.d. https://www.nyenrichmentgroup.com/nutrition-education-for-parents.

Savage, Jennifer S., Jennifer Orlet Fisher, and Leann L. Birch. “Parental Influence on Eating Behavior: Conception to Adolescence.” The Journal of Law Medicine & Ethics 35, no. 1 (January 1, 2007): 22–34. https://doi.org/10.1111/j.1748-720x.2007.00111.x.

Momwithfive, "Tips How to Celebrate Health and Wellnes Milestones (2023)," Mom With Five, September 26, 2023, https://www.momwithfive.com/en/2023/09/25/family-celebration-healt-wellness-milestones/.

Printed in Dunstable, United Kingdom

71297579R00117